FROM
DAYLIGHT
TO
DARK

Finding Work in an Inaccessible World

Valerie D. Maidment

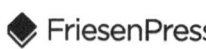 FriesenPress

One Printers Way
Altona, MB R0G 0B0
Canada

www.friesenpress.com

ISBN
978-1-03-830428-5 (Hardcover)
978-1-03-830427-8 (Paperback)
978-1-03-830429-2 (eBook)

1. HEALTH & FITNESS, VISION

Distributed to the trade by The Ingram Book Company

Dedications

I dedicate this book to all people who are blind or visually impaired. Since losing my vision suddenly in 2008 I have learned through experience what a blind person has to go through, the barriers and discrimination faced on a daily basis. I want to change what it is to be blind today. I hope this book will help people see what we face and maybe take the step to breaking down barriers and making things more accessible for all.

Many thanks to my friend/coach, Sharon LeShane without whom I would not have written this book. I never thought I could write a book but Sharon told me I could and encouraged me to do so and now here it is. I hope you enjoy reading it.

A big thank you to my girls, Kelsey and Alyssa who helped with choosing the cover for my book. You were a great help, without you both I would not have been able to do it myself.

Last but not least, my husband Wally who stuck with me through it all. We both had a big ordeal to go through. and it wasn't easy. I don't know if anyone else would have stuck by my side as he did. He was always there when I needed him.

Table of Contents

Introduction

Vision loss or blindness can affect anyone at any time. It can happen suddenly or gradually over time, depending on the cause. No matter how it originated or the timeline, vision loss changes a person's life drastically, and it can affect one's quality of life, independence, and mobility. Everything changes; a person has to start all over again when vision is lost later in life. They have to learn new ways to do everything. They are no longer self-sufficient. No matter how independent a person thinks they have become after losing their sight, there is always something they will need help with.

So when someone loses their vision, it also has a significant impact on their family and friends. For example, having to depend on someone to take them to an appointment, or even just to the mall. The family member or friend has to take time out of their day to help. They may not mind, but it still affects them. Wherever visually impaired people go, people around them feel like they are responsible for them, making sure they know where they are going and that they don't have an accident and hurt themselves.

The complete loss or deterioration of existing eyesight can feel frightening and overwhelming. It's not easy for someone to know their vision is getting worse every day, and that there will come a time when they cannot see. This leaves them wondering about their ability to maintain their independence, pay for needed medical care, retain employment, and provide for themselves and their family.

Finding employment with vision loss is not an easy task, as you will see from my experiences throughout this book. Employers don't want to hire people with vision loss; they are afraid we may get injured or need some help; they don't know how to associate with a blind person; or they just don't want to be bothered. From my work experience, it seems that larger companies or organizations hire people just so they can say they are inclusive, when all you are to them is a number. They want to make it look good for themselves but will not completely accommodate a person.

These are situations people with vision loss have to face on a daily basis. Why businesses that can afford it can't make their workplace accessible, I can't understand. We want to be able to work as well as everyone else. Everyone has to make money to live. Personally, if I cannot go to work and fully complete what it is that I am hired to do, I don't want to be there. I want to work, not just be a number.

Activities most people take for granted present barriers to Canadians who are blind or visually impaired. These obstacles can be found in our physical infrastructure, education and healthcare system, the job market, social function, and individual attitudes and expectations. It first starts with the ability to get around. Not all buildings and structures are accessible, thus limiting where people can go and where they can't. If buildings are not made accessible, it makes it harder for a person to find a job or go to school.

Next comes social isolation. If buildings are inaccessible to the blind community, it affects how we are able to socialize with the outside world, and this in turn will lead to anxiety and depression. The economic impact of vision loss is also substantial. If a person can't get an education to allow them to find work, and they are discriminated against by employers, how can they afford to live? This in turn reduces a person's quality of life. The barriers a blind person can come up against are endless. It takes someone strong to be able to cope with everything.

The biggest hurdle to overcome with vision loss is finding a job. In Canada, the unemployment rate for people with sight loss is 14.5 percent, which is three times higher than the general unemployment rate.[1] For some reason, employers are not interested in hiring a person who is blind. Despite having comparable or higher qualifications than their sighted peers, people with sight loss face significant challenges when it comes to joining and staying in the workforce.

In my opinion, people who are blind are looked upon as not being able to do anything. As a former executive member of a non-profit organization, I felt left out. I told my fellow executives if they wanted me to do anything to let me know, and if I could do it, I would. If I wasn't able to do it, I would tell them. I wanted to be considered as part of the committee. However, this didn't happen. I was still left out.

I don't understand how we are looked upon like this. People have to realize that we learn to do things in a different way. We want to be included, not just pushed to the side. For those who believe we are not capable of living as independently as everyone else, spend some time with a blind person, and you will find out what we can do.

I have had people ask me, "How do you do this?" or "How can you remember the way to get this done?" It's not something I think about; it's just a part of completing a task and of trying to live as independently as everyone else. We learn to do things in ways sighted people would never come up with. Vision loss enables us to look at things differently

---

1   MacNeil, "Let's Boost the Employment Rate for Canadians with Sight Loss."

and figure out how we can get things done. Technology is advancing every day, allowing the blind to live more independently.

Learning to cope with vision loss isn't easy, and we go through many ups and downs. It is an emotional battle trying to live our life. Some people cope with it well; however, there are those who just want to give up. I am not one of these people. I hope you will join me on my journey; this book will allow you to see how vision loss can change a person's life, but if you are willing to give it all you've got, not letting anyone or anything hold you back, you will be able to live as independently as others.

Chapter 1:
Waking Up to Vision Loss

I was born on November 6, 1969, at the Dr. A.A. Wilkinson Memorial Hospital, in Old Perlican, Newfoundland and Labrador, Canada. Old Perlican is nine kilometres from Bay de Verde, where my parents, Shawn and Louise Broaders, lived. I had two younger brothers, Shawn Jr. and Darryl, who was the youngest. Mom had a miscarriage before I was born, and I had another brother who passed away shortly after he was born.

Bay de Verde is a small fishing community that depends on the fishery for their livelihood. Most everyone who lived in Bay de Verde either fished out of the harbour or worked at the Quinlan's plant. Bay de Verde is located at the tip of the Bay de Verde Peninsula. We lived in a small two-bedroom house just up from the Anglican church. My father fished with my grandfather, James Broaders.

When I was only a few weeks old, my parents took me for my checkup and found out I had a condition called hydrocephalus. This is a disorder in which there is a buildup of cerebrospinal fluid around the brain that typically causes increased pressure inside the skull. The pressure from too much cerebrospinal fluid can damage brain tissue and cause a range of impairments in brain function. It can occur at any age but is commonly found in infants and adults sixty and over.

My parents were shocked. They could not believe it. They had not seen any symptoms, but the doctor noticed it immediately. Apparently, my head was bigger than normal for a child my age.

I had to have surgery to relieve the pressure around my brain that was causing my head to swell. I was to have a shunt inserted into my skull to drain the excess fluid from my brain. This would be done through a tube going into my stomach. The surgery was done by Dr. Maroon, and it went well. Luckily, I did not have any brain damage. I spent a week in the Janeway Child Health Centre in St. John's, Newfoundland and Labrador. This hospital was for children sixteen and under. After I was released, I had to have regular checkups to make sure everything was working properly and there was no buildup of fluid.

My surgery didn't stop me. I grew up doing most everything a child my age would. When I was two, we moved from Bay de Verde to Mount Pearl, a city near St. John's, so my dad could be closer to his new job at CIP Containers, a company that made boxes for almost everything. I loved my dad's job; he would bring home cardboard for me to draw on. There was cardboard all over the house.

I remember living in a basement apartment; I could not see out the windows, so I would stand up on the back of the chesterfield to look out. Mom didn't like this because she was afraid that I would fall and hurt my head. At the end of the street where I lived was a convenience store, and when Mom and I would go there, I would always get a Pixy Stix. It was my favourite treat, and I looked forward to going to the store to get one.

I started school at age four because my birthday was in November. I didn't like school much, and for the first year I missed many days, probably because on December second of that year, my baby brother Shawn was born, and I wanted to stay home to be with him.

I attended Mary Queen of the World School in Mount Pearl. I can't remember much about it, but one thing does stand out. I recall standing outside my classroom by the coat racks and just down the hall was a cafeteria full of people. I know that because there was a window in the door, and I could see them. What I was doing or why I was there I don't know, but it sticks out in my mind. I guess I was afraid to go in with everyone.

At the end of the school year, my teacher did not want to pass me because I had missed so many days. She told my parents I had not attended enough classes to know the work. They wanted me to do kindergarten over again. My parents were not satisfied with this, so the principal agreed to put me in Grade One halfway through the next year. However, this did not happen, and I did two years of kindergarten. After this, my parents decided to move back to Lower Island Cove, where my grandparents on my mother's side, Charles and Florence Fagner, lived. It had nothing to do with my doing two years of kindergarten; my parents just decided they wanted to move back home.

When school began again, my parents registered me for Jackson Walsh Elementary in Western Bay, about thirty minutes from Lower Island Cove. I travelled by bus to and from school each day. I remember my first day of Grade One clearly. All of my classmates were sitting on the floor in front of our teacher, Mrs. Baggs. I recall her asking me to stand up and tell everyone my name and where I lived. I stood up and did as she asked.

This time, I did enjoy going to school each day and interacting with my friends, and I had no trouble. The only thing I didn't like was not being able to take part in gym class, for fear of hitting my head. Still, Grades One and Two went well, and my medical checkups were good.

I was now in Grade Three and still liked going to school. I was fond of my teacher, Mrs. Gladys LeShane. She also lived In Lower Island Cove with her husband, Ken, who was the postmaster. Then one day that year, it happened again: my shunt was blocked. I had to have surgery to replace it. I don't remember much from this time, but everything went well. I spent about a week at the Janeway in St. John's.

After I was released, I found out that my teacher had sent home my homework for every day I was in hospital; I had lots to do, as I had to catch up on everything before I returned to school. When I did return, all of my friends and my teacher were happy to see me.

I continued with my regular checkups, and all of my follow-up appointments went well. There was no buildup of fluid, and I was doing fine in school. Then one day during a checkup, my parents and I got a surprise. My doctor told us that everything was working as it should, and I did not need the shunt anymore. However, Dr. Maroon said he wanted to leave it there in case there came a time when I did need it.

I continued on through school with no issues, graduating and moving on to college. I completed a bookkeeper-clerk course at the Avalon Community College, as it was known then, now College of the North Atlantic or CONA. For about the first month, I boarded in a home just up from the college, but I was homesick. Luckily, I was able to find a couple of fellow students, Jim and Joey, who drove me back and forth each day. It didn't matter what the weather was like; we made it to school every day.

The next year, I completed a computerized accounting course at Keyin Technical College. I had trouble finding transportation to and from this program, though. There was a bus operated by the Squires in Sibley's Cove that would travel to St. John's on Monday, Wednesday, and Friday. I took the bus to Carbonear, got off at the end of the road, and walked down to the school. I managed to find a way there on the days when the bus wasn't running. I did miss a few days, but I made it through the program.

After college, I spent my time looking for work. I almost got a job doing bookkeeping; I had an interview in St. John's, and it went well. The owner told me he would have hired me, but because he did not know enough about bookkeeping himself, he would not be able to help me out if I got in trouble.

During this time, while babysitting for a friend, I met my boyfriend, Wally. He was from Bay de Verde. Each day when I was babysitting, Wally would show up. I got to know him and looked forward to seeing him. One night in November 1989, we went out, and our relationship officially began. When we had been together for a while, I moved in with him and his sister, Nellie. They had another sister, Dulcie, who lived in St. John's, and two brothers, Archibald, who lived in Toronto, and Arthur, who lived in Toronto but moved back to Botwood, NL with his girlfriend when he retired. They also had a brother, Robert, who passed away at an early age. They lost their mom when they were very young, and their father passed away about ten months after we met. After moving in with Wally, I went to work in the Quinlan Brothers crab plant.

Wally and I were together for about three years when I became pregnant with my daughter, Kelsey. She was born on May 24, 1993, at the Carbonear General Hospital. I took the next season off from the crab plant; I wanted to look after my daughter. Wally and I enjoyed raising Kelsey; it was a new experience for both of us.

My friend Serena's mom had a convenience store in Bay de Verde. She had offered me a job, but after discussing it with Wally, we agreed that I would make more in the plant. When Kelsey was almost four, I was offered a position working in a convenience store in Lower Island Cove, where I grew up. I knew the owners; they were the aunt and uncle of my friend, Sandi. Sandi and I spent a lot of time together throughout high school, going to the game room in Job's Cove on the weekend. This was our regular hangout.

This time, I accepted the job and gave up working in the plant. I enjoyed working at the store and getting to know everyone. After being there for a year, my second daughter, Alyssa, was born on August 10, 1998. I took the next year off to care for my children. When I returned to work, it was only in the evening from five to ten, which worked out for me; I was able to care for my girls during the day and their father looked after them until I got home at night. I travelled back and forth over the barrens—the area between Bay de Verde and Old Perlican. This can be a rough region at times, especially during the winter months.

I continued to work at the convenience store for the next seven years, getting to know the owners well. Then one day they announced that they were going to retire, and they were putting the business up for sale. I enjoyed working there and did not want to give it up. I wondered if this was something I would be able to do. After some consideration, I decided I wanted to buy it for myself. When the owners decided on a price, I went and got the loan to purchase the store; my journey into entrepreneurship began. After all the papers were signed and everything was ready, I took over the business in August 2004. For the first little while, I ran the store by myself, spending the whole day there. I had Wally, and even sometimes my girls, help me out whenever they could.

I travelled from Bay de Verde to Lower Island Cove on a daily basis to run my business. There was a small apartment attached to the store, and there were times during the winter when we would stay there. The store was about twenty kilometres one way from my home in Bay de Verde. I still travelled the barrens in all kinds of weather, from bright sunshiny days to the middle of a winter blizzard. This was my least favourite time, as I could not see a hand before me, let alone one behind me. Most of the time, I drove myself to work, but when it was really bad, I would get Wally to take me and come back to pick me up.

We continued to do this for a number of years. Then in 2007, Wally and I decided it was time to move closer to the business, figuring it would make things a little easier. We purchased a house in Lower Island Cove and moved up there. Kelsey, Alyssa and even Nellie were excited; they were going to be moving into a new home, and it was close to my parents.

Once we settled in, there were renovations that I wanted to do, which took up all of my time. Between running the store and looking after my girls—Kelsey was fourteen and Alyssa was nine—I had a number of things I wanted to get done. There were windows that needed to be replaced, painting to be done, and we had to install a rail going up the stairs. Wally and my dad, Shawn, were kept very busy.

With moving in and the renovation work being done, the house was a mess; everything was everywhere, and I could not find anything. The girls were picking out colours for their bedrooms. I thought we would never get it done, but eventually, we did—just in time for Christmas. The girls were getting excited for Santa and wanted to start decorating the house and putting up the tree.

It was early in December, and I was not feeling well. I was having headaches between my eyes, and it hurt to tip my head back. I was thinking it was my sinuses; it was normal for me to have a sinus infection. I had been back and forth to the doctor, but it didn't seem to be getting any better. I was taking medication and using nasal spray.

On Christmas Eve, I had an appointment with an ENT specialist in Carbonear. My father took me because Wally was helping out at the store; it was very busy at this time of year. The specialist could not find anything wrong. He gave me another prescription for my sinuses, and we came back home. By the time we got there, I had a headache. Thinking it might be a migraine, I went in to use the bathroom, closing the door and turning off the light to see if it would help. The next thing I knew, Nellie was calling out my name and trying to get me up off the bathroom floor. I had passed out.

Nellie called Wally at the store. When he got to the house, he suggested I go to the emergency room in Old Perlican. The doctor on call checked me out and could not find anything wrong, so I was sent home again. The next day was Christmas, and I started to notice my vision wasn't the same. I contacted my doctor, who told me it may be a side effect from the medication I was on, so I stopped taking it. I made it through Christmas without having to go to the hospital, but I wasn't feeling any better.

Then one night, early in the new year, I woke up and the left side of my mouth had gone crooked. I did not know what was going on; I was thinking I was having a stroke. I was scared; I woke Wally and told him what was happening. We headed back to the ER in Carbonear. This hospital, approximately forty minutes up from Lower Island Cove, is the main facility outside of St. John's to go to for treatment. Most everything that can be done in St. John's can be done in Carbonear.

While there, I had a CT scan done to check my head. I was told that my shunt was blocked, and I would need surgery to correct it. Here

I was, thirty-seven, and I needed to have surgery again after all these years. I could not believe it. The last time it was checked, everything was working on its own.

We were going to have to go to the hospital in St. John's. Wally and I went back home to let Nellie and the girls know what was going on, and then we got ready to go to the city. When we arrived, I went to emergency and was admitted. After being in the hospital for a few days, having many tests done and explaining my history with hydrocephalus, nothing was done; I didn't have surgery. The doctor who had put in the shunt when I was a baby, Dr. Maroon, was there. I recall him saying that he remembered the shape of my face, so he also knew my history.

One of the tests I had done at this time included lying on a table while fluid was taken from my shunt and then put back again. The purpose of this examination was to see if the shunt was working. The fluid was inserted, and I was told to lie still. I did this for a while, and then I was asked to move my body to see if the fluid would drain down into my stomach. I did as I was told, but nothing happened. This went on for a while, and then I was sent back to my room. Thinking back, this was a sure sign that the shunt was not working properly. If it was, I should not have had to move my body; fluid would have just gone through the tube and into my stomach. I should not have to jump up and down to get things to work.

There were a few more tests done, and then one night the doctor came into my room. He looked into my eyes and asked a few questions, and then he told Wally and I that I had a "slight case" of multiple sclerosis (MS). I did not know what to think; I didn't even really know what it was. As Wally and I did not know anything about MS, we took the doctor at his word. Exactly what he meant by a "slight" case, I don't know.

Multiple sclerosis is a disease that impacts the brain, spinal cord, and optic nerves, which make up the central nervous system and controls everything we do. The exact cause of MS is unknown, but we do know that something triggers the immune system to attack the CNS.[2] The resulting damage to myelin, the protective layer insulating wire-like nerve fibres, disrupts signals to and from the brain. This causes unpredictable symptoms such as numbness, tingling, mood changes, memory problems, pain, fatigue, blindness and/or paralysis.[3] Everyone's experience with MS is different, and these losses may be temporary or long-lasting. Here I thought I was going to have surgery.

The doctor told us he was going to give me a treatment, and it would probably be a while before I needed another one. Wally and I were surprised to hear this, as we were told the shunt was blocked and that I needed surgery. We did not know what to believe, but we figured the doctor was right. After all, he was the doctor. The treatment consisted of steroids by IV, two hours a night for five nights.

Each night after my treatment, Wally and I looked forward to having some time alone. He stayed with me through it all, sleeping in a chair by my bed. We would listen to the radio station CHVO, which was located in Carbonear. At this time, they were changing over to a new name; it was going to be known as Kixx Country.

I took all the treatments and was then told I could go home. However, just before I was to be released, I had a seizure—or so we thought. After having a test done, I was informed it was a really bad anxiety attack. Wally had been sent out of the room, and he said that

---

2   Mayo Clinic, "Multiple Sclerosis."

3   National Multiple Sclerosis Society, "Myelin and Multiple Sclerosis."

from where he was standing outside the door, he could see that there was froth coming out of my mouth, and my eyes were rolled up in my head. Wally was scared. He did not know what was happening to me. I didn't know what was going on either. I didn't have anything like it before, but they still released me. My brother, Shawn, came to pick us up, and we went home.

Here I was at home and not feeling much better. My vision was almost gone. As we were not given any info on MS, we assumed this was how I was supposed to be. I thought it was just a side effect. By this time, all I could do was get from the bed to the recliner and back. I started to have seizures. At first, they were rare, but they did get more frequent. When I would take with a seizure, my oldest daughter, Kelsey, would sit by my side and hold my hand until I came out of it. But my youngest, Alyssa would run off to her room. I guess this was her way of dealing with it. It had to be scary for both of them.

We still thought this was how MS was supposed to be. Then about three weeks later, Wally was helping me out of the tub and the side of my face started to swell up. He got me out and went downstairs; by this time the swelling had gone down. However, it didn't stay this way for long. It occurred again and again until I became afraid and wanted to know what was going on. I called my family doctor, and he suggested I go back to the hospital. I called in, but the doctor who diagnosed me wasn't on call that weekend. I didn't like hearing this. I wanted to see the one who treated me, not someone else.

The swelling did not stop, and I wanted to know what was happening to me, so I decided to go back to the hospital. I saw a different physician this time. We had to wait a while to see him, as it was a Friday, but eventually I got in. Wally wheeled me into his office; I was in a wheelchair because I could not stand up. The doctor asked me a few questions, including whether or not I had had a spinal tap. I told him I had not; I had different tests done, but no spinal tap, which he found hard to believe. He then looked into my eyes and told me I didn't have MS, I had pressure, and it was because the shunt was blocked. Then he informed me that I needed to have surgery to correct it. He then ordered a spinal tap and went home for the day.

The nurse did the tap; Wally was there. The nurse could not believe it; she had never seen pressure like it before. The next morning, the doctor came back to see me. He also could not believe the amount of pressure; he performed an additional tap, then told me I needed surgery. The nurses got me ready, and the next thing I knew, I was being rolled into the operating room.

I remember opening my eyes and wondering where I was for a few seconds. Then it came back: I had been taken to surgery to have my shunt replaced. I felt relieved it was over. I was in recovery, and I felt very warm, as I was wrapped in heated blankets. I could hear the nurses talking but all I could see were shadows; I could not pick out what anything was. I would not have been able to tell where I was but for the noises.

The nurse came over and wanted to know how I was feeling. The first thing I asked her was what the time was. She told me, and she said that my father had called several times to see if I was out of surgery and how I was doing. I told the nurse that was like my dad. He was impatient. She told me I had to stay in recovery for another while, and then they would take me back to my room. I relaxed and fell back to sleep.

The next thing I knew, I was being rolled off the elevator and into my room. The first thing I heard was Wally's voice. I was so happy to hear him, and he was glad to see me. He had spent the time in my room waiting for my surgery to be over.

The nurses lifted me off the stretcher and put me on my bed. They asked if everything was okay, and then they left. By this time, Wally was over by my side. He was happy the surgery was finished. We spoke for a while, and then he let me rest.

That night I did not sleep very well. I suddenly woke from my sleep. I was feeling anxious, and my heart was beating very fast. I guess this is what caused me to wake up. I think I may have been having a panic or anxiety attack. I just didn't feel good. I then remembered where I was and what I had done. The right side of my head was bandaged up, and I was afraid to move it. Wally never left my side. He stuck with me through all the ups and downs. If it had been anyone else, they would have probably packed up and left. Even though we had been together for almost nineteen years at this time, neither one of us had thought about getting married.

The next morning, I woke up early. I was hungry and could not wait to have breakfast. When food arrived, the nurse put up my bed and pulled up my tray. As I could not see, Wally helped me. At this time, my vision was almost completely gone, and I did not know what was going to happen. Wally would put my food on the fork or spoon and give it to me. I was extremely glad to have him there, as I would not have been able to do anything on my own. This made me think, *What am I going to do? Am I going to be able to manage this? Will I be able to take care of myself? Is my vision going to return?* It was all new to me; I never dreamed I would go blind. As a child, I was not too fond of the dark.

I still did not know what was going to happen. Nobody said anything about my vision before surgery, and they still had not. Their focus was replacing the shunt and getting the pressure down. I would not find out anything until I saw my ophthalmologist. I was thinking that the return of my vision would depend on how much damage was done from the pressure on my optic nerves.

Wally helped me with everything. He would even help me get to the bathroom. This would have been hard for me by myself. I did not know where anything was and could not see where to go or what I should do. I thought to myself, *How am I going to be able to do anything again? I am going to be dependent on someone else.* This was not me; I was used to doing things independently.

After a couple of days, I was able to get up and sit in the chair. Wally would take me for a walk through the corridor. It was good to be able to walk without pain. I could not see much. It was only when someone or something moved that I would notice it. Wally took me by my arm and guided me so I would not run into anything. We went to the end of the hall, where there was a large window overlooking the parking lot. I remember gazing out, seeing what looked to me like a day obscured by fog. This was not actually what the day was like, Wally told me it was a clear day, and the sun was shining. This is how my vision was now, and I was hoping it would eventually get better.

Finally, the day came when I was released. I was so excited to be getting out of the hospital. I wanted to get back home, but I wondered, *What now? Am I going to get my vision back?* It was going to be a waiting game.

Chapter 2:
Depression, Anxiety, and Vision Loss

As a child, I experienced anxiety and depression. I did not know what it was or why I was feeling this way; I just knew it was different. I would tell my parents, but they would just tell me it was nothing. I do not blame them for how they managed the way I was feeling. Back then, there was hardly any talk about mental health. If someone was dealing with a mental health issue, it would be kept secret.

I remember going shopping with Mom when I was around ten and having to leave the store. I was feeling different and could not stay there. I could not explain how I felt. We left, but Mom did not understand. She would say, "Don't be silly; it's nothing." At this time, I thought she was right. I did not know what was happening to me. I just knew how I was feeling. In retrospect, I would say I was either having a panic or anxiety attack. Once I got out of the store, I felt better.

When I was in elementary school, I would have panic attacks if I was sitting in the middle of the classroom. Back then, I did not know what was happening to me. I would get my teacher to let me sit by the window and open it; I would then feel okay. The music room at our school was in the middle of the building, where there were no windows, and I would have to ask the teacher to let me sit by the door. I know this sounds silly but at the time it wasn't silly to me. It is only now that I am an adult and have learned about anxiety and panic attacks that I understand what I was feeling at such a young age.

I continued having anxiety and depression throughout school. Sometimes it would seem like it was gone, but it would always come back again. I still had not told anyone about it. I did not know what was going on, and I was afraid of what people would think of me.

While attending college in 1989, I dealt with depression. I managed to continue with my studies, though, and it gave me something to focus on. I made it through and graduated. I found that I would be depressed for a while and then it would be gone, and I was feeling more like myself. Then when I lost my vision, I had reason to be depressed again. Being able to see one day and not the next can affect a person's mental health.

Researchers estimate that between a quarter and a third of adults with low vision or vision loss experience depression or anxiety.[4] This is understandable, as everything changes for them. It makes a person feel different. They feel like someone who needs help, has lost their independence, confidence, and self-worth, and is disconnected from friends. These feelings can worsen once a person realizes they cannot do the things they did before. Just imagine the anxiety you would feel if you were told you were going to lose your vision. How would you deal with it? What would you do? How would it make you feel?

The first steps in getting help for depression can be hard. You do not want anyone else to know how you are feeling. At first, you may deny that things are different, or you may feel helpless. You may not know what help is available, what services are right for you, or how to access them. Be honest with yourself and reach out to a friend you can trust.

---

4   Grassnickle, "Your Mental Health: How Vision Loss Impacts Depression."

Then find a mental health provider in your area that can help you. Remember that depression and anxiety are treatable. Medication, talk therapy, and self-guided learning can all be effective. You don't have to go through it alone.

Chapter 3:
Returning Home

Here I was back home, and it was so good. It was even better that I had no pain, but my face was still out of shape from the former pressure. I was feeling more like myself, but I could still not see. I could not wait to see the ophthalmologist. I wanted to know when my vision would return. I wanted to see what he would tell me. At this time, I could not do anything. It was all new to me, and I didn't know what I was supposed to do. At first, all I did was sit around in my recliner, except when I had to go to the bathroom or eat. Mealtime was different, as I could not tell where my plate was or what was on it. Someone would have to tell me where things were. For example, potatoes on the left, chicken on the right.

I also had to learn to get around my home. I knew the layout, but I had to come up with a way to know where I was. I ended up following along the walls and furniture to get where I wanted to go. My home was a two-storey, so there were stairs. Wally had rails installed. I would hold onto both rails and count the stairs as I went up or down. This way I knew when I reached the bottom or top.

I had been home for about a week, when my stitches were to come out. The public health nurse showed up early that day. I was nervous; I thought it was going to hurt, but it just tickled. The scar started about two inches above the top of my right ear and went down behind it, all the way to my earlobe. I don't remember how many stitches there were. Now that my hair was down, the scar and missing hair didn't look too bad. I had long hair, but they only shaved under it, and you could not even tell I had had anything done.

Finally, the day came when I was to see the ophthalmologist. I was excited. Everything looked fine; the pressure was going down slowly. However, my optic nerves didn't look good, because of the extended pressure. The doctor said that he could not tell me if I would regain my sight or not. He told me my optic nerves looked like those of a dead person, and he could not say if they would regenerate or not. Then he informed me that if any vision came back, it would probably take a year or so. He also questioned why I did not have surgery earlier, explaining to Wally and I that when I saw him in the hospital the first time, he had written down on my chart that the shunt must not be working. Did my doctor read the chart? I still had no idea how this had all happened.

I was disappointed; this was not what I wanted to hear. Now I had to continue to learn to live with vision loss, while hoping I would get some sight back. This was not an easy task. I did not know what to do or how to do things. I had wanted to be told that my vision would eventually return.

What was I supposed to do now? My life as I knew it had changed. It was a struggle trying to figure out what I could do and how to do it. Just thinking I would not be able to see again was unbearable. I could not think of it. I had to take it day by day and hope my vision would return; without this hope, I would not have been able to cope. All I could do was wonder if things would have been different if I had had surgery earlier. There would not have been so much damage done to my optic nerve, and maybe it would have been able to regenerate. After coming home from the hospital the first time, I was worse than when I went in. I was having seizures, could hardly stand up, and had trouble keeping food down. I lost twenty-five pounds.

It was now early February 2008. I was starting to feel and look more like myself every day. The pressure was going down, and my face was returning to normal. Still, my vision had not returned.

Although I had people around me, I felt alone. I was the one with vision loss, and it made me feel left out. My family would go about their normal day, and here I was, left alone, not knowing what to do next or how I would learn to cope with not being able to see. It was going to take some time to get used to vision loss, while hoping it would return. I was going to have to learn to do things all over again, and I had no idea where to start.

My girls knew what was going on and that I did not know if my vision would come back. They were there to help me; however, at first, it seemed like my youngest daughter, Alyssa, didn't want me to use my white cane. When we would go out, she would come up with some reason why I should not use it. I guess she didn't like me being seen with it, but after a while, she came to terms with it. I began to use the cane regularly.

There were days when I felt like I was trapped, especially when I would wake up and my vision was not the same as it was the day before. This is a result of the kind of vision loss I have. My doctor told me that no two days would be alike. With the optic nerve continuously trying to regenerate, my vision was always changing. One day it was darker, and then another day I would only see out of a small hole, and the next day the hole might be bigger. It was continuously evolving. This is something I had to learn to deal with. It wasn't easy, and some days were better than others. It was frustrating; it made me feel more trapped and more dependent, not being able to do things how and when I wanted.

I wasn't used to having to rely on others; I felt that just because my life had changed, it didn't mean that my family's also had to change. I didn't expect them to stop what they were doing for me. However, I did know that they would be there if I needed them. I knew I couldn't depend on other people to be by my side all the time. I had to learn to do things on my own, one way or another.

Then one day, I had had enough; I wanted to do something. I decided it was time for me to get back to living my life, even if I only started out small. After all, if you want to get somewhere, you can't just give up. Anyone who knew me knew I was not a person who was satisfied just lying around the house. Before losing my vision, I was always on the go. I didn't stop, but I loved it.

I remember being bored one day, and this brought me to my first task. I had Nellie put my clothes in the washer and dryer for me, and then I folded them. This was a simple job, but at least it was a start. It didn't take much to fold laundry. I just picked up the item and lined the ends up, folded it one way, and then lined it up again and folded it the other way. I had someone bring the basket of clothes to me so that I would not have to carry it while navigating my home.

I did this on a regular basis, but it still wasn't enough for me. I had always been active before losing my vision. The next chore I took on was drying dishes and putting them away. Another simple task. This wasn't too hard, as I knew the layout of my kitchen and where everything went. I used the countertop to guide me along. I found the right door by counting them, and then I opened the door and felt around to find the spot to put the dish.

This went on for six weeks until my recuperation from surgery was over. I was restless and wanted to do something more. It was then I decided I wanted to go down to my store. I wanted to get out of the house and see what was going on.

This made a big difference. First, I got to visit with my friends, who I considered to be a part of my family. I missed them, and they missed me. As time went on, I started doing little things. I would get one of my employees to put the sticker in the pricing gun, and then I would price groceries and put them on the shelf. They would show me where to put it, and then I would line the items up and stack them on the shelf. Eventually, I started to check out a few things. I had no trouble doing this because I knew the prices of everything, and I knew the buttons on the cash register. I could do it from memory.

With a little help, I made this work. The help I got was from my family and employees; the doctor and hospital didn't have anything to do with it at all. Everything I did I figured out a way to do it myself. I would even bag groceries. I then started going to the store every day, as I had before my vision loss. It was great to get back into a routine. I now depended on the store. It was what I looked forward to every day, just being able to get out of the house and mix with people.

For the first little while, when Wally and I went shopping, I would wait in the car and not go in. I am not sure if it was because I could not see to get around or just because I wasn't ready. I was still learning to deal with my vision loss, and I guess I was afraid. I didn't want to knock anything down or run into anything. It was also different being out in public and not being able to see who was around or what was going on. I had to depend on what I was hearing. This continued to be my way of life. I just didn't know what to do or how to go about doing things. There were many times when I would think to myself, *What if*

I don't get my sight back? I would think about the things I would not be able to do and see.

I would go upstairs at night and lie on the bed and just think. There were many times when I would break down and cry. I wondered why this was happening to me. It was something I did not understand. I knew people had it harder than I did, but I was still struggling to deal with what was going on. It took a while, but I managed to cope with it a little more each day, especially when I would learn a new way to do something. I was still hoping I would get some vision back, and I still do every day. This will not stop.

After a while, I managed to regain a little vision in my left eye, but the right one remained the same. I had what sight I was going to get back by this time.

I tried to figure out what I was going to do now. *How am I going to learn to do things on my own?* I knew the Canadian National Institute for the Blind (CNIB) was there for people like me, but I wondered what they could do. Then one day I decided I wanted to find out.

I went to visit them; they were very welcoming. The first thing we did was take my picture for my CNIB ID card. This card showed I was a member. There was someone there for everything a person may need. While there, they showed me different types of technology that were used to help a person read. There were things as small as a magnifier and as big as a closed-circuit television (CCTV).

I tried various magnifiers to see what worked best for me. I was excited. I found one that I could use with the vision I had in my left eye. It would be slow, but I could manage to read. The CNIB had a program where they would loan clients items to try out to help them decide if they wanted to purchase them. This allowed me to use devices for a couple of weeks to make sure they were going to work for me.

I used the magnifier and loved it. It allowed me to read things; however, it took me a while. I didn't mind, as now I was able to read on my own. I was even able to find the numbers on a bingo card. Our volunteer fire department had a weekly bingo game on TV, and now I was able to play again. My magnifier allowed me to go down through each number to see if I had the one called. I only had one card, so this made it easier for me.

I purchased this magnifier, and I used it up until a few months ago, when it finally gave out; I had it for about twelve years. This was the first of many things I used with vision loss. I wanted to replace it, but this one wasn't available anymore. There were many different magnifiers to choose from, but I could not find one that helped me the way this one did, and there was no way to fix it.

Wally's other sister, Dulcie, lived in St. John's. We did not hear from her very often. Occasionally, she would call, and then other times, we would reach out to her. One day a friend told Wally that Dulcie was in the hospital. She hadn't told us. I called the hospital and confirmed she was there. The next day, we went in to visit her. We wanted to find out what was wrong.

It turned out that she had cancer and was going to have to have treatments. At this time, she was living by herself. Wally decided this was not going to work; he wasn't going to let her go through this by herself. In April 2010, she moved in with us; now we had a full house. Dulcie enjoyed being with us. There wasn't much that I could do for her at the time, but she was happy to just have someone around to talk to. I did make something for us to eat occasionally, though.

Dulcie wasn't well. She had good days and bad days. She continued with her treatments. Things went okay for the next couple of months. Then one day in July, she was at the hospital to get her treatment but couldn't get it. Her bloodwork wasn't as it should be. She was then admitted to hospital.

For the next few weeks, it was back and forth to the Carbonear hospital to visit her. She kept asking us when she was going to get to go home, and we could not tell her. We just did not know. In early August, they moved her down to the hospital in Old Perlican. This made it easier for us to visit her. We were there every night.

One night, I decided to stay home and let Wally go. The next morning, on August 18, 2010, at about six-thirty, the nurse called and told us that Dulcie had passed away. In the next few days, her older brothers, Arch and Arthur, and her sister-in-law, Wanda, came home for the funeral. All the family was shocked; nobody knew she was sick or having any problems. Wally had a hard time believing it; it all happened so fast. Dulcie's life was in St. John's, and she had never kept in touch. It was only by accident one day we heard that she was in hospital, and now she was gone.

Chapter 4:
Wrong or Right?

There was this older lady, Florence Snelgrove—known to everyone as Miss Florence—who would come to the store occasionally; I knew her all my life. She was a quiet and very friendly person, very mild-mannered, and everyone got along with her. She and her husband, Cliff, had had a store in Lower Island Cove. I went to school with their daughter, who was also named Florence. My friends and I would hang out at the store every weekend.

Each time Miss Florence dropped by for something, she would tell me not to let it go. She said that what the doctors had done to me wasn't right, and they should be made aware of it. Since she had known me since I was a child, she knew my history. Everyone in the community had heard I was diagnosed and treated for MS, but that it had turned out I had pressure from the shunt being blocked; this had delayed me from having the surgery done sooner, which may have prevented my vision loss.

This got me wondering, as I thought the same thing. I decided I was going to investigate my options. I visited a few lawyers, and they told me they thought I had a case. They knew from what I had told them that it was a misdiagnosis because the doctors knew my history, the CT scan at Carbonear hospital had shown the shunt was blocked, and the ophthalmologist had even written it on my chart. What happened, I will never know, but something or someone wasn't right. However, the lawyers I visited did not take on malpractice cases. I would have to find one who did. I did not give up; I kept looking for an attorney to take my case.

Finally, one day, I went to Gittens and Associates in St. John's. The lawyer I was meeting with was Ernest Gittens. Wally and I went into his office and sat down. I told him my story, and he listened carefully. After finishing, I asked him if he thought I had a case. He said that I did, and I cried. Knowing what I went through and having someone else agree with me was validating. It hurt to know that my vision loss could have possibly been prevented if surgery had been done earlier.

Ernest told me my first step would be to get a doctor from outside the province to review all my files. This would give us the actual proof we needed to go ahead with the case. I found a doctor from Ontario who was willing to do it and had my files sent to him.

It was some time before he got back to us. This wasn't an easy task; he had to go over every little detail in my file. However, when he finally contacted us, the results were not good. He had found that there wasn't only one mistake made but many. This again made me break down and cry, knowing what had been done to me. I had my daughter, Kelsey, read the letter he wrote to me, and I could not believe it. Could this have been prevented? Why were there several mistakes? Not considering the CT scan done at the Carbonear hospital, not doing a spinal tap when they knew my history, not considering what the ophthalmologist had written on my chart, and not realizing my shunt was blocked by the test I had done, when the fluid did not run from my shunt into my stomach. Was this real, and why did it happen? This is a question only the doctors can answer. They were given my history and even had the CT scan from Carbonear hospital, and they still misdiagnosed me.

The next step was to file the papers against the doctors, and yes, there was more than one involved; the physician who reviewed my files had listed three. Once they were served the papers, the process had begun. Now we just had to wait to see what they were going to do.

I continued to help at the store. I was there every day. Things were going well, but my vision had not returned. My younger brother, Darryl, would spend a lot of time just hanging out. He would help whenever there was something to do. This I appreciated, as I could not do things like I used to.

Then one day, Dad called and said that he had to take Darryl to the hospital. They were in Carbonear shopping, and Darryl wasn't feeling well. They took him over to emergency. This was on a Tuesday afternoon. The doctors ran some tests and found out he had bleeding ulcers. They gave him the treatment he needed, and he was doing well. I was up to visit him, and he was able to get out of bed. He was to be released in a couple of days.

Then on Saturday night, after Wally and I came home, we found out that Dad had called. I was wondering what was going on; it was late for him to be phoning. I decided to call him back. It was then that he told me Darryl wasn't doing well and was probably going to have to have surgery. With that, Wally and I left for the hospital, but not before calling Aunt Mary. I wanted to let her know what was going on and ask her if she could come to the hospital. I figured Dad would need someone. Mom was there, but she was in shock. She could not believe what was happening. She just sat there and didn't say anything.

We arrived at the hospital about thirty minutes later, and just after we got there, Aunt Mary showed up. They had taken Darryl down to surgery. After a while, his doctor came up to explain what was going on. She informed us that Darryl had a lot of little pinholes in his stomach that were bleeding as well. This is what was causing the trouble. The bleeding was coming from everywhere, making it harder to repair.

During surgery they had to send to St. John's for platelets, and in this time, Darryl's heart stopped. The doctors got him back. When they got the platelets, they finished up the surgery. This was about two in the morning. The doctor told us that the surgery was over, but Darryl wasn't out of the woods yet. We would now have to wait to see what would happen.

Wally and I got ready to go home, and Aunt Mary left with us. Mom and Dad were going to leave after they had seen Darryl. (Dad later said that after getting to see him, Darryl didn't look good.) We came home and went to bed. The next morning, at around seven o'clock, we awoke to the ringing of the phone; it was Dad telling us the hospital had called them, and Darryl wasn't going to make it.

I could not believe my ears. This could not be true. Dad and my brother, Shawn, left and went to the hospital. Mom was just not able to go. Dad and Shawn made it just before Darryl passed away. When I got there, he was gone. My heart was broken. I didn't know what to do. I went in to see him, but I had to leave. I touched his arm and ran out. I broke down crying. My little brother was gone, and so fast. It was hard to believe. He was only thirty-four.

The next few days were hard, preparing for the funeral and picking out a casket. Dad took care of everything. I did not go to help pick out the casket, as I would not be able to see it, so I had him describe it to me.

Darryl had died on October 3, 2010; Mom and Dad's anniversary was on the fourth, and Mom's birthday was on the sixth. Dad did not want the funeral until after Mom's birthday, so it was held on October seventh. It was a hard day on everyone. Mom and I were still in shock. Mom could not even look at him. At the funeral home, she agreed to go into the room, but she wanted the casket closed. This is what we did for about half an hour, when there was only family there. She didn't have much to say, and then she went home, before the service started.

Dad was finding it hard to believe his youngest son was gone. It was a shock for everyone. He was so young. Darryl was the type of person who did not want to bother anyone else. If he had a problem, he would deal with it on his own and not tell anyone. It made us wonder if he had not been feeling well but did not want to bother us. He spent his time at home just hanging out when he wasn't working.

Chapter 5:
Next Steps

Eventually, things started to get back to a new normal, or something that resembled "normal." Life would never really be normal again; Mom and Dad were lost. They still hadn't gotten over the shock. It was hard for them to believe that their youngest son was gone, and so unexpectedly.

The house was empty; Darryl had lived with Mom and Dad. He spent most of his time at home, except when he was working at the plant or when there was a dance at the community centre in Lower Island Cove. It was known as the Association for Youth and Leisure Time Activities. This community centre held events for both the young and old. He loved going to the dances and listening to the music. He and his buddy, Russell, very seldom missed a dance. They would be the first there and the last to leave. Outside of work, Darryl would be with Mom and Dad wherever they went. He would even take Mom to things when Dad didn't want to go. They spent a lot of time going places just for the ride, and to get out of the house.

I continued to go to the store every day, but things were not the same. My brother was gone. When I would walk into the store, I missed him. He would always be there. It was hard to believe and even harder to get used to. It took a while, but eventually things started to feel a little better. There were times when it was very busy, and then times when it was very quiet. We were nearing Christmas, the busiest time of year other than summer. Everyone was getting ready, shopping for things they needed. The snow had started to fall, and the ground was turning white.

The kids loved it. They were getting ready for the annual Santa Claus parade put on by the community centre. It was a big day for everyone. After the parade, it was back to the building for refreshments and photos with Santa. There would even be a tune or two from the Cadets, after which they would be on their way to another parade. They were in demand, especially this time of year. The kids had a blast, eating hot dogs, having their picture taken, and just running around, letting off steam. The next morning was a breakfast with Santa, another favourite for the kids, and even some adults.

Still, with Darryl gone, things had changed. He always looked forward to Christmas, especially having turkey. He enjoyed putting up the tree just to be able to sit back and look at the lights, which he spent many hours doing. Then, of course, he anticipated the New Year's Eve ball. He and his friend would be the first ones there. Darryl loved the music, but it was hard to get him to dance.

With the first holiday season without Darryl behind us, I started to think about my business. I was wondering if I could continue with it or not. Everything had changed; my vision was gone, and so was my brother. This was a lot of adapting for me. What was I going to do? It was getting harder for me to keep control of the business. Could I sell it, and did I really want to? I spent many days and nights trying to figure out what I was going to do. If I sold it, what else would I do?

After much consideration, I decided it was time. As much as I loved it, I had to give it up, so I put it up for sale. It was not what I really wanted to do, but under the circumstances, I did not have much choice. I couldn't look after it the way I had. I wasn't always sure what was going on. Week after week, it seemed like I was ordering more stock than the business was selling. It didn't seem to be busy during some weeks, but for some reason I would have to order the same as I did the week before. I began to wonder what could be going out without my knowing about it. I was not able to do the bookwork, and I had to depend on one of my employees. This wasn't a good way to have a business. I was new to vision loss and didn't have the knowledge and technology to help. The store needed more attention than I was able to give it at that time.

It was for sale for about eight months without any offers. There were a couple of people who inquired about the price, but nothing came of it. I was ready to give it up; I didn't want the responsibility, and the enjoyment was gone. I was worried that it wouldn't sell, as it was a difficult time of year.

Then one day a local resident of Lower Island Cove came along with an offer. The papers were drawn up, signed, and everything was legal. Within the next two weeks, in January 2011, there were new owners. I had worked with vision loss for three years, but I now accepted that it was too much for me. I was sad to see it go; the store was like family to me. I knew most of my customers, and we had developed great relationships. This is what I was going to miss the most, getting to see and chat with them every day. The day came, and I passed over the keys and walked out, wondering what I was going to do next.

Some days it would be okay to get out, and others it would not. I spent a lot of time at home. The weeks and months passed slowly for me, and I was still wondering what to do next. I was missing the shop in one way, and in another way, I wasn't. It was the people I missed the most.

Staying at home most of the time was getting to be boring, but I didn't know what to do with myself. The only time I would get out would be when we went to Carbonear for groceries or to go down to visit Mom and Dad. I had too much time on my hands; I had to find something else to do. This was not me. Anyone who knew me knew I could not stop; I was always going somewhere or doing something. I was not content staying around the house all day. Vision loss had slowed me down; I didn't know if I was going to get past it.

There wasn't much for me to do, but for my oldest daughter, Kelsey, there was lots. She was about to graduate from high school. It was now May 2011, and they were getting ready for graduation night. The gym was decorated, and everything was ready to go. Kelsey was all dressed up in her prom dress. This was a very special night for her. Wally and I were so proud of her.

This is one of the things that vision loss has taken from me: I was unable to see how beautiful my daughter was and watch her as she walked upon the stage to accept her diploma. Then it was her dance with her father. The only thing I could do was listen to the music and try to imagine what they looked like. They could describe it all they wanted, but it would not take the place of being able to see it with my own eyes.

After some time, I decided to see if I could find a job. There had to be organizations that would assist me in trying to obtain employment. I kept calling places I had been told would probably be able to help, but I had no luck.

Then one day, I finally found someone; it was the Canadian Paraplegic Association, who I learned helped people with physical disabilities find work. I made an appointment with them to meet and discuss my options.

Our meeting went very well; I had found a great place. However, it was going to take some time for me to find a job. I would have to find an available position and bring it back to them. They would then intervene on my behalf, working with the employer to see if I would be qualified. The problem was, there wasn't much available where I lived. I would have to look outside of the area, and this was probably going to take some time.

I didn't give up; I made it my mission to find a job. I kept looking for appropriate positions every day. Then, after a few months of searching, I thought I had found one. It was at Old Perlican Terrace, the old age home in that community. I had been talking with the manager, and she agreed to hire me. At first, I was told the position was there for me, but they were not able to tell me when it would start. I was disappointed. I waited and waited. Then one day, they called and asked if I would be able to come in. They set up an appointment for me. I was excited. This was going to be my first job after losing my vision and giving up my business.

However, it did not turn out as I had hoped. When I got there, they told me that funding had run out, and they would not be able to hire me at this time. This was another big disappointment. All I could think of was that I had to start looking again.

After getting over this setback, I started to look again. I searched and searched, with no luck. I would find something, but it would not be for me, or it would be too far for me to travel. I was looking for something that was closer to my home, as I would have to get Wally to take me back and forth. This went on for some time. I remained home, bored, with nothing to do most of the time. I spent my days folding clothes and washing dishes. I wanted to get out and mix with people. I wanted to have someone to talk to.

Then one day out of the blue, in the middle of January 2015, I had a call to come in for an interview. It was with Old Perlican Terrace, the old age home that could not hire me before. I was so excited. After spending so much time in the house, I was eager to get out with people.

I told Wally the minute I got called that he would have to take me there for the interview the next day. I was asked a few questions, and they explained what I was going to be doing and how this program, sponsored by the Canadian Paraplegic Association, worked. If a business was willing to hire a person with a disability, they would pay a percentage of the hourly rate for several weeks in the hope that the person would be hired on permanently. They told me everything was a go, and they would be in touch with the start date.

I was thrilled. I was finally going to get out of the house and interact with people. I would be working alongside the residents as a personal care attendant while getting to know the staff. This is what I was looking forward to. I was to start in a couple of weeks.

But before this could happen, the orientation and mobility specialist from CNIB had to come out and go through the building with me, making sure things were safe and helping me learn how to navigate. I was scared and excited; excited to have found a job but scared because I did not know what to expect. This was my first time in the work force since losing my vision. Was I going to be able to do it? Was I going to be able to navigate the building by myself, or would I get lost? All these thoughts and many more went through my mind.

The day the orientation and mobility specialist came out, I was ready. I had decided that I was going to do it. We went through the whole building. She taught me how to use my white cane to get through the hallway. She showed me ways to figure out where I was and gave me tips on how to use my cane. There were little things I used to identify where I was. She also had a meeting with the staff. There were things they needed to know to assist me while working there. For example, if I was in a room and someone entered, they would have to let me know they were there and when they left. It was a great day learning how to navigate the building. Now, was I ready to do it by myself? I would soon find out. I had to start working the next day.

At the time, there were approximately twenty residents living there. There were some I did not know, but there were others I did. One of them was a great aunt on my father's side. She was ninety years old at the time and has since passed away. There was also a lady from the town I grew up in and knew quite well. Most of the residents were from communities in the surrounding area. While I was unfamiliar with some of them, they had been told about me, and they were excited to have someone there to keep them company and help them out when they needed it. They were also looking forward to having events to participate in as well.

My workdays consisted of washing and folding clothes; this was something I had learned to do at home. Vacuuming and cleaning tables was also part of my job. Because I had a little sight, I would be able to see the edges of a mat and the table. This allowed me to complete these tasks.

The ladies looked forward to a game of bingo every day, but we could not get the men to join in; they would say it wasn't for them. I had the bingo numbers written on pieces of cardboard with a black marker. This allowed me to call the numbers because now I was able to read them.

On sunny days, we would go out for a walk around the building. This is where the residents helped me. I would walk alongside them, and they led the way. I kept them company, and they guided me around the parking lot.

The highlight of the week was when a musician or band would come in to play for them. I would check with talented musicians from the local communities each week to see if they would come and entertain the residents; they loved to hear the music and sing along with the songs. There were even a few brave souls who would get up to dance. One of them was my aunt Mary; she loved her music and dances. She was not a resident of the home; everyone was welcome. They all had a wonderful time and looked forward to the next one. It kept me busy trying to find musicians to play for them. Each day, Wally would drop me off, then pick me up in the afternoon. Occasionally, when Wally couldn't come, my aunt Mary would drive me home. All I had to do was call her, and she would be there.

I had been working there for almost two months, when my mom fell and broke her shoulder. Wally, Mom, Dad, and I had been to Carbonear and were on the way home. Mom wanted to drop in to a friend's house before we went home. It was March, and there was still slush and snow on the ground. She got out of the truck and as she went around it, she slipped and fell. Wally helped her up, and she said she was okay.

Her shoulder hurt the next day. Dad took her to see the family doctor, who did an X-ray and told them that she had crushed her shoulder and was going to need surgery. This was on Wednesday, and surgery would be on Friday. On Friday morning, Mom, Dad and I got ready and went to the Health Sciences Centre in St. John's. Dad had to drive, as my brother, Shawn, was working. I took the day off and went in with her and Dad. It's times like this when I felt like I should be doing more. If I was able to see, I would be able to drive them to town and give Mom the help she would need after surgery. I would also be able to help her after the operation, as once they put in a plate, she would not be able to lift her arm over her head.

Mom went into surgery. We were told it would not be long. Dad and I stayed in the waiting room. It took longer than anticipated; I was starting to wonder why.

Finally, the procedure was over, and Mom was doing well. She had been moved upstairs to a room. We went up to see her. She was doing fine, with only a little pain. They had put in a plate because the bone had been crushed. She was expecting to get released the next day. Dad and I left to go home. I told her I would talk to her in the morning before I went to work.

The next morning, I called, and she was doing well. I told her I would call her again after work. Dad and Kelsey went in to see her. Shawn was already in town. Mom was doing well but did not get out that day. Just before supper, Kelsey and Dad left to go home.

Shawn was working and living in the city at the time, so he was there to visit Mom again that night. This was on a Saturday. However, before Dad and Kelsey reached home, my brother called and told me that the nurse had called him, and Mom had gone into cardiac arrest. She was unresponsive.

I was in disbelief; she was fine when I was talking with her in the morning. Now I had to tell Dad and Kelsey; I didn't know how they were going to react. I decided to call Aunt Mary and see if she would go up to the house to tell Dad, and I would wait for Kelsey. He was shocked, as he had just been with her, and she was fine. He helped her get ready for supper before he left. My brother went back to the hospital that night; Dad and I waited to go in the next morning. She remained stable overnight.

The next morning, we walked into the room and there she was, lying in the bed with her eyes closed. We went over to her and spoke, but we got no response. Dad even took her hand, and there was still no response. I spoke to her, but still nothing. We stayed there for most of the day. My youngest daughter, Alyssa, came to see her. She spoke to her, too, but still got no response.

At supper time, we left to go home. Nothing had changed all day, and everything remained the same overnight. Mom was still the same the next day. She was on life support and was too unstable to move. We had no idea why this had happened. After discussing her condition with the doctor, we had a hard decision to make. It didn't seem like she was going to make it. What were we supposed to do? Were we ready to take her off life support?

After much discussion, we decided to do what we knew Mom would want. She would not want to be kept on life support. Hard as it was, we knew what we had to do. Dad had decided it was the right thing.

We informed the doctor of our decision. Shortly after, they were there to disconnect her. We were all in the room as the doctor unplugged her life support. Dad saw her take her last breath. He said to the doctor, "She is gone, isn't she?" But the doctor said her heart was still beating. In a matter of seconds, it stopped, and she was really gone. It was so hard to believe. She was only sixty-six.

The next few days were hard on Dad and everyone else. He had to prepare for her funeral. I helped where I could, but my vision loss made things difficult. She passed away on Monday, March 30, 2015, and was buried the following Thursday, just before Good Friday and

Easter. I remember it was a cold, windy, and snowy day. I wondered how we were going to move on from this. It was such a shock.

After Easter, I returned to work. However, it was not the same. All I could think of was Mom. Mother's Day came and went. I had arranged for some music for the residents. All the mothers had a great day.

The next couple of months went by slowly. The manager told me that I was not going to be hired permanently. There wasn't a position there for me after the program was over, which was at the end of July. I guess I was lucky to have gotten hired for as long as I did. They may have created the position so I would get some work, and so they would get some help that did not cost them as much.

However, there was now a reason to look forward to the end of my contract. I still wanted to find the perfect job, but I needed the time off for a reason that I had been keeping secret: Wally and I had finally decided to get married, after all these years. We agreed we would not tell anyone right away; we wanted to keep it to ourselves for a while.

I never thought we would marry; we were young when we got together, and it never came up. But when I brought it up after Mom's death, Wally had been thinking the same thing. I think Mom's accident may have given both of us some perspective. After being together for twenty-six years and having two girls, we both wanted the same thing. It was time.

We had decided to get married on August fifteenth. This meant it was going to be a rush. We didn't want a big wedding, just a few friends and family, but by the time we finished up, we had a few more. Altogether there were around twenty-five guests. I had my uncle, Lee Broaders, providing the music, and our friends, Bertha and Boyd King, were going to be our witnesses.

The next couple of weeks were very busy as we got everything ready. We had to get the rings, and as I was not able to see them, I had my daughter, Kelsey, describe them to me as best as she could. After feeling the stones in the ring, I decided on the one I wanted. I also had to get a dress and find someone to marry us. I picked out my dress more by how it felt than how it looked.

We got Reverend Cruthers from the Anglican Church in Bay de Verde to marry us. We decided we were going to get married at the house, and my cousin, Christine, had volunteered her new home for a small reception. It was just down the road from where we lived. Shawn's girlfriend helped with the decorating; everything looked beautiful. The day had arrived quickly. The girls were getting excited. Everything had all come together. Christine's house was decorated beautifully, and all was ready at our home.

I was getting a little nervous. Bertha, Boyd, and Dad were there, then the rest of the guests started to show up. The wedding was to start at seven p.m. I was upstairs getting dressed. My aunts, Mary and Nita, were helping me out. We were having a ball trying to get the strings in my dress tied. It took a little while, but we finally got it done. I was hoping it would not come untied during the service.

It was then time. I had to walk down the stairs to where I would meet Dad. He was waiting at the bottom. He then walked me over to where Wally and the reverend were waiting. Lee was singing and everything was quiet, except for the sound of a couple of people shedding a few tears. The service began.

The wedding went off without a hitch. The ceremony was short. The book was signed. Pictures were taken, and then we left to go to Christine's house. The reception was small and simple. There was plenty of food and drink. The reverend and his wife even stayed for a while. My uncle sang my favourite song, "Walk Through This World with Me" by George Jones, for our first waltz. Reverend Cruthers sang "Amazing Grace." It was beautiful; he did an excellent job with it. The night was full of laughter, food, and fun. It was a special time for us.

Chapter 6:
Returning to School

It was now May 2016, and my baby, Alyssa, was about to graduate from high school. This was a very exciting time for her; however, once again it was sad for me. Here was my second daughter graduating, and I had to go through the same thing as I did with Kelsey, not being able to see how beautiful she looked in her dress and how special it was when she danced with her father.

The next few months were more of what I was used to—doing daily chores and being bored—except now I was a married woman. I still missed working; I really wanted something else to do. My lawsuit had been ongoing; I had been to several discoveries. A discovery is a meeting between both parties to obtain additional information for the case. Then one day, I got a call from my attorney. We were going to meet with the doctors' lawyers to see if we could get a settlement without going to trial (which had been scheduled for early October 2016). This I was not looking forward to. It would bring back memories of what I went through.

I had been considering going back to school for some time. I would think to myself, *Yes, I think I will,* and then, *No, maybe not.* I wasn't sure if I would be able to do it; it was going to be different with vision loss. This went on for a while; I would go back and forth with my decision.

I could not decide what I wanted to do or if this was something I was willing to take on. I knew it wasn't going to be easy.

Finally, one day, I decided I was going to take a chance and do it. *Why not? I have nothing to lose.* I applied for the Office Technology program at Keyin College in Carbonear, the same school I had attended after graduating high school. I chose this program because I thought I would like to get a job as a receptionist or secretary. I knew I would enjoy interacting with people, and I had several years' experience with customer service. It would also allow me to brush up on my accounting skills.

I was accepted, and the fact that I would be a student again became real for me. I was going back to school. I could not believe it. This was around April 2016. The first thing I had to do was learn how to use a computer while being visually impaired. At this time, I didn't have much experience with them anyway, so I was going to have to learn regardless.

Being a member of the CNIB, I knew most everyone who worked there. I had collaborated with Jason Rose on a few little things. I knew he had trained for different types of technology. Jason has only 10 percent vision himself. He told me I could do it; I was a quick learner.

We connected, and he got me using a computer with NonVisual Desktop Access (NVDA), which is a free screen reader available with Microsoft that is used by blind/visually impaired people; it reads the text on the screen aloud, enabling people with vision loss to use the computer. Once he got me going, he figured out what I would need to get through the program. The biggest and most important item I needed was a screen reader.

He figured NVDA may not have all the features I needed, so he suggested Job Access with Speech (JAWS), a screen reader that lets visually impaired or blind people listen to the text on a screen. It provides both braille and speech output that greatly benefits those with impaired vision. This assistive technology allows the blind community to be able to work.

The next thing I needed was textbooks. They had to be purchased in audio format, and they would have to be ordered by the school. I contacted the principal at Keyin College, and she ordered them for me. The audio books cost me the same as the textbooks would have, plus I got a copy of the actual textbook, which would come in handy if something had to be checked on.

Jason told me I was going to need a Victor Reader Stream. This is a handheld, pocket-sized digital media player that allows the blind to listen to audio books, podcasts, newspapers, web radio, and music wherever they are. It is also great for taking notes or recording lectures. It has a tactile interface that makes it easy to use.

The Victor Stream was my go-to. I used it for everything. I took notes, recorded classes, and was able to listen to my textbooks. Once we had figured out what I needed, we got down to work. We spent many hours working together and making sure I knew how to use the screen reader. It was difficult at first, but I managed to get the hang of it. With this program, there were different keyboard shortcuts that allowed me to perform the same functions as a person using a mouse would. These shortcuts would take me to where I wanted to go.

The day came when Jason and I both figured I was ready. It was time to test out what I had learned. It was off to school for me. My cousin was attending Keyin at the same time, so we travelled back and forth together.

However, before I could start, an orientation and mobility specialist would have to come out from the CNIB. At this time, it was Alice.

Together with the principal, we went through the school. I learned how to navigate with my white cane and learned the route to take to each of my classes.

Alice gave the principal suggestions on what she could do to make the school more accessible for me. Some things that had to be done included putting a special kind of tape at the top of the stairs and on the steps. I was able to use this tape to tell when I was getting close to the top of the stairs. With the little vision I had, I was able to pick out darker colours, which helped me to get around. This didn't take long, as the school was still located in the same building where I had attended after graduating from high school. I remembered my way around. With this all taken care of, the next thing to do was to get started.

The first day came, and I was nervous. I hadn't been in a school in a while, and this time, I was visually impaired. I started to second guess myself and began to wonder if I was going to be able to do this. Here I was in a place where I did not know anyone. The first few weeks were a little difficult, getting used to using the computer, JAWS, and just navigating the building.

It was a learning experience for my instructor, Steve, as well as for myself. If I didn't know something, he would look up to see if there was a way to complete the task. Together, we made it work. If we came across something that didn't work, we would figure out another way to get it done. In most cases, we were able to get through it; however, sometimes, we did not. I was new to the technology and was still trying to figure it all out. There were times I just had to reach out to Jason to see what he thought. Looking back now, I realize there was much more to JAWS than I knew about. If I had to go back to school today, there would be things I would be able to do that I could not before.

Jason was a great help. What he didn't know he also researched for us. It would take me longer to complete exams, so I was not in the same room as my fellow students. The principal allowed me to do my exams in an office connected to hers. This way I would not interrupt anyone. I was excited to be able to keep up with the rest of my peers. I met many new people. Some were just out of high school, and others were around my age.

I met Joyce and Lori, who both had children as well. They were also looking to further their education and get back into the workforce. We got to know each other quite well, spending hours in the lunchroom going over the classes and assignments we had. Some of them were harder and more complicated than others. But for the most part, they were quite accessible. I managed to get enough information to be able to understand the course.

There was only one class that wasn't accessible: Simply Accounting. The program was not made accessible for JAWS, and there were parts of it that the screen reader would not read, with no way to access the information through keyboard shortcuts. This surprised me because this accounting program was around when I attended college in 1989. Here it was, 2016, and it still had not been made accessible.

The time had come. In early October, I had to take a day off school to go to town to see what was going to happen with my lawsuit. We were going to see if we could get a settlement out of court. We all met in the boardroom. Wally wasn't allowed to go in, so he waited outside. The lawyers were talking back and forth, and I listened carefully. This went on for a while, and it seemed like we were going to have to go to trial.

We took a break and then went back. With much more discussion, they finally came to an agreement. My lawyer, Ernest, got what he was looking for, so it was over. The doctors agreed to settle out of court. Once again, I broke down and cried. I guess it was knowing that the doctors were admitting defeat, and that what they had done was wrong.

My program was normally eight months, though I did it in twelve. I did not do all the courses that were required in one semester. The principal had agreed it would make it easier for me if I didn't have too many courses to focus on at the one time, as there were times when it took me longer to complete a task.

When December came, I was getting close to the end of the first semester and exams. This was a nerve-racking time. I wondered if I was going to be able to do it. It was twice as hard for me, as I not only needed to know the material covered in the course, but also how to navigate JAWS to get it done. Trying to study and make sure I knew how to navigate the programs was stressful. If I did not know how to use the technology, there was no way I was going to be able to get it done.

It was going to take more time for me to finish my exams. Some days it took longer to finish than others, but I made it through. I passed all my exams. I did quite well and was very pleased with myself. For people who are visually impaired, the simplest things we learn to do on our own make us feel good. It's a feeling like no other. Almost like winning the lottery.

Next, it was on to the second term. Some of the courses continued over into the new semester, and there were new ones I had to start. Once again, my instructor and I came together to make things work. My friends and I continued to help each other when there was a lot of work to be done. I spent many hours a night working through it. It was all worthwhile. I was enjoying it. Time went quickly. The next thing I knew, it was the end of the second semester and the end of the program for my friends. Everyone did well on their exams, and it was off to graduation for them in April. My friends were ready to move on to their work term. This was not so for me. I had another semester to complete.

The third semester started for me, but it wasn't quite the same. My friends were not there, and there were new people who had started. I felt a little alone at first. However, by now I was familiar with the program and found it much easier.

I spent many hours reading and working hard. I really wanted to finish this program so I could get out and look for work. This was my goal: to find a job. By now I was looking forward to my own graduation. My last semester was a little lighter, as I did not have as many courses as I did in the previous two semesters. Little by little and bit by bit, I got through it. It was exam time again, and I did well.

Finally, graduation day came, and Wally and the girls were there. I felt so good going across the stage to accept my diploma. I had done it, even with my vision loss. It gave me a great feeling to have accomplished something on my own. It's milestones like this one that make a person feel good.

Next, it was time for my work term. At first, I thought I was going to be doing it in Carbonear at the Advanced Education Skills and Labour office as it was then known. But the principal decided that it would be better for me to go to the city and do it. The place they decided on was Empower, The Disability Resource Centre. I think it had to do with my vision loss, and this organization helps anyone who has a disability. Empower gives people the opportunity to socialize, assists with finding a job, helps them advocate for themselves, and learn how to use different types of technology that can improve their lives. They also work with employers who are interested in hiring people with disabilities. Empower also holds weekly activities, and they even plant a vegetable garden each year, picking the crop and planning a meal in the fall. Everyone comes together for some food and fun.

During my work term at Empower, I was responsible for answering calls and transferring them to the appropriate department or taking messages as well as collecting and delivering mail to the staff. I enjoyed my time there, and I got the opportunity to learn things while getting to know many people.

I remember one situation in particular. One day this older lady came in, and she was very upset. She told me she had a bad experience with one of the Go Bus drivers and wanted to report it. I told her I would see what I could do. I reached out to the manager and explained the circumstances, and she told me where to direct the lady. I told her and then sent her into the office. When she came out, she was much happier. She thanked me for assisting her. It was a great feeling knowing I was able to do something to help.

I spent the four weeks of my work term with my daughter, Alyssa; she was attending university at this time. I would get the Go Bus in the morning and then again in the evening. The Go Bus is a taxi for people with disabilities. They pick you up and drop you off where you want to go. It can be a taxicab, or a bus used by those in wheelchairs. It is an inexpensive way for people with a disability to get around and feel more independent.

The month went quickly, and then I returned home. Now it was time to look for a job. This wasn't going to be easy living in such a small community. The population for Lower Island Cove, according to the 2016 Canadian census, was 245.[5] It only had a post office,

---

5   Government of Newfoundland and Labrador "Lower Island Cove Profile"

a convenience store, and a gas bar. I would have to go outside my community to Carbonear—population 4858, according to the same census[6]—to try to find work, and it still wasn't plentiful there.

As I mentioned in chapter 5, the community centre in Lower Island Cove was known as The Association for Youth and Leisure Time Activities, or 'The AYLA' for short. The late Peter Bursey started the AYLA in 1989. It served the communities of Job's Cove, Lower Island Cove, and Caplin Cove. It was a place to offer programs and activities for the children in the area. When the 'youngsters' did not have something going on, the public could book the building for birthday parties, showers, and weddings. Every August, they would hold the annual regatta. This consisted of a folk festival, boat races, games of chance, local entertainment, and fireworks. To end off the regatta, there was a dance. Everyone looked forward to it each year.

The AYLA had an executive committee. There was an annual general meeting (AGM) each year to elect new members. Just before the annual meeting in 2017, I was asked if I would like to run for secretary. I thought about it and decided to give it a try. I was elected at the AGM. I was looking forward to taking on something new. I was to take minutes, help with the planning of meetings, advertise and help plan events, and take care of any correspondence and activities.

I would record the meetings on my Victor Reader, then before the next meeting, I would go back to the recorded meeting and type up the minutes. This I had done on my computer with the help of my screen reader, JAWS. Then at the next meeting, I would listen to my screen reader and read out the minutes. We had meetings at least once a month for the public and the executive committee when needed.

---

6   Government of Canada, Statistics Canada. "Census Profile, 2016 Census Carbonear, Newfoundland and Labrador."

I was there to help, but I felt left out at times. I think people thought I couldn't do much. Sadly, this is the reality for people who are visually impaired. We are looked upon as not being able to do anything. It's the first thing people think of when they hear a person is blind. This may have been the case years ago, but with technology today, things have changed. We can still do things; we just have a different way of doing them.

During one of the executive meetings, I decided to speak up for myself. I told the committee I was there to help in any way possible. If they needed me to do something, they could just ask. If I could do it, I would. There was always a way to figure things out. This, unfortunately, didn't change much. Occasionally, I would be asked to do something, but not as much as I would have liked. I spent three years on the committee and then decided it was time to give it up. I was ready to move on.

Chapter 7:
From Unemployment to Entrepreneurship

The job hunt was not going well. I spent a lot of time looking but could not find anything. Employment postings didn't come along very often where I was living. Then one day, I came across one for a bookkeeper. Now that was me! That was something I could do. I love bookkeeping. Working with numbers is my passion. I did all the bookkeeping for the business I had to give up.

I sent in my resume and was excited to get an interview. I did not disclose my disability. Wally took me, and I went in using my cane. Of course, this showed them I was visually impaired.

The bookkeeping job was with a garage located in Harbour Grace. The mechanic's secretary was the one to do the interview. The mechanic himself was also there. I thought the interview was going quite well. I was qualified to do what they were asking. At the end, she told me she had more people to interview. I asked if I would be notified as to whether or not I was successful, and she told me I would. She said that whether or not I got the job, I would be called by Monday. The interview was on a Friday.

I was excited. I was hoping to get the job. I waited and waited patiently until Monday. Monday came and went, and I still had not heard back from her. It didn't look good. I was hoping to get a call, but it never happened. Not even to let me know I didn't get the job, after telling me she would call either way. I didn't like or appreciate this. I don't think it was right. I also believe that her decision was made the minute I walked in the door with a disability. You can almost see the change in the interviewer when a person comes in. The way they conduct the interview is different. I can't explain it, but I can usually tell the outcome.

It is discouraging when this happens but, unfortunately, it does, and more often than you would think. It makes a person feel left out. Unfortunately, the sad reality is that there are people who look upon the visually impaired/blind in that way. We may be more qualified than the other people interviewed, but we still will not get the job. Why employers look at us differently, I can't understand. It's not fair, but it happens. I personally think employers are afraid to hire people like us. This causes a person to lose confidence in themselves and sometimes give up. It hurts, but I was not going to let it stop me. I wanted work, and I was going to find it.

A few months later, I came across a position with Empower, The Disability Resource Centre, where I had completed my work term. They were looking for an Independent Living (IL) intern. This position consisted of promoting their programs and services, and the work was to be done while working for another employer. Its purpose was to get employers to hire people with disabilities and hopefully get them into the workforce. It was two jobs in one.

I met with them, and they told me if I could find some organization or business willing to hire me, I would get the job. It did not have to be a business; it could be a community centre or non-profit organization.

Whoever hired me would also benefit because I would be doing work for them but getting paid by Empower.

I decided to approach the AYLA community centre, where I had worked as a secretary. Maybe there were things I could do for them. The committee discussed it and agreed I could work from there. I was excited to get started.

Before I began, I had to go to town for a week of training. People from other parts of the province also attended. However, I was the only blind person. Therefore, things were not set up to accommodate me. For example, we had to make a slide show, and this was not something I had a lot of experience with. I didn't know how I was supposed to present one, not being able to read my slides.

During this week, we learned what our responsibilities were and what was required of us. When the training was completed, I returned home to start work at AYLA, where I was a member of the executive for three years. My duties included completing any tasks required for the building, researching for programs and grants, writing correspondence, creating the monthly newsletter, and taking calls. In my spare time, I was responsible for promoting the programs offered by Empower.

A client from Mariner Resource Opportunities Network (MRON) was also working at AYLA. His name was Christopher. MRON is an organization that helps people with intellectual disabilities find employment. People hired by MRON would have a coach working with them most of the time. Christopher had a coach from Lower Island Cove, whose name was Ann LeShane. They were responsible for cleaning up after events held at the centre plus any other things that needed to be done. I worked from the office while they worked in different areas of the building.

Throughout my contract with Empower, I would hold workshops at various places, promoting the programs and services in the Trinity/Conception area, as there was no office there. Occasionally, I would go out to the mall or some other business to set up a display. I would send emails out to the schools to inform them of the programs available through Empower. If they wanted to know more, they would reach out to me, and I would go to the school and do a workshop for them, explaining in more detail the programs that were available.

I worked with them for eight months. During this time, Ann LeShane and I became friends. We had known each other before, as she was married to a man from my hometown. She would go with me when I had a workshop. She was a great help to me, especially with setting up the tables and getting everything ready. There were times when she would give me a ride as well. We would have many chats about everything. She even made dinner for us on my birthday. I finished up in March, and she and Christopher finished up a little earlier. A while after they were finished, she found out she had cancer. She passed away in November 2019.

Once again, I was unemployed. I started thinking, *What can I do? I want to work but can't find employment that will last for long.*

I then had an idea. I had done accounting when I graduated from high school and then again in 2016, when I went back to school with my vision loss. I knew how to navigate the programs, so why not start my own bookkeeping business?

I had heard of the Community Business Development Corporation (CBDC). This is an organization that helps people who want to start a business. They offer many services to get a person started. I submitted my application for service and was approved. Then I had meetings to attend and got signed up with the program. I also had to attend some workshops, which taught participants what was involved in running a business.

I got my office ready and purchased the equipment and programs I needed. One of these programs was Quick Books, which is best known for its bookkeeping software; it has a desktop and online version. The great thing about this program was that it was accessible for me. It was just what I needed to get my business going.

In late July 2019, my business was launched. I called it V & M Bookkeeping Services. The V and M were my initials, which I used to give it a personal touch. It was time to see how this would take off. It was slow going at first. My first client was a patron of CBDC; I met her and her husband while attending workshops there. They were just starting a business and were looking for a bookkeeper. I was excited; I had my first client. This was my passion. I loved doing book work and was looking forward to helping and getting to know these people. After all, they were willing to give me a chance, and for that I was very grateful.

I spent much of my time the next few months marketing and looking for clients. I found a few; however, they were only one-time clients. I wasn't going to get my business off the ground this way. I continued to search, but it wasn't looking prosperous. It seemed like there wasn't anyone out there looking for a bookkeeper.

I was getting disappointed. Most of the people I spoke to with a business were doing their own books. Once again, I was left being bored. I had lots of extra time on my hands.

I then decided I wanted to volunteer my time. Tammy Bursey was now the owner of the store I had sold. I approached her to ask if there was any work I could do to help. She told me she would think about it and get back to me. The next week, she contacted me. She wanted me to come to work on Wednesday and Friday mornings to help with the inventory that was coming in. I would stock shelves and coolers and help with the dishes in the kitchen. Tammy's mom was there every day making homemade food to sell. I was very grateful that Tammy gave me a chance to show her what I could do. Not many people would do this for a blind person. I very much appreciated it. I continued to volunteer there for over a year.

With V & M Bookkeeping Services not doing well, I decided to go another route. Maybe I could do tax returns. I was going to hire someone to do tax returns for me; this would give me time to learn how to do taxes myself and find out if the tax programs were accessible for me to use.

I put an ad on Facebook. A few people applied, but they were not what I was looking for. Then one day, I got a call from a woman inquiring about the tax preparer position. I interviewed her and found out she had been an employee with Revenue Canada. She was now retired and looking to do tax returns herself.

I could not believe it. This was just what I was looking for. I decided to hire her. The next step was to get set up. I had to apply for the Studio tax program so we would be able to e-file the returns. Once this was taken care of, we decided how much to charge for the returns. We didn't want to be too expensive but still wanted to make money. Once we decided on an amount, I started advertising on Facebook. It took a little while, but then the clients started showing up. The business was picking up. However, this didn't last very long. It all came to a stop suddenly.

There had been an infectious disease called COVID-19 spreading around the world. It had reached Canada, but it had not yet reached Newfoundland and Labrador, and everyone was hoping that it would not. Wally and I were out celebrating St. Patrick's Day in March 2020. There was a lot of talk about it. Everyone was worried what would happen if it reached Newfoundland and Labrador. People were dying all over the world. There was no cure for this disease.

That night after getting home, Nellie told us the unfortunate news: there was a case found in Newfoundland. This was when everything turned upside down. The next few weeks were chaos. Everything was shut down. People were not allowed to leave their homes. Schools, restaurants, businesses that did not carry grocery items, and any building that held functions were not allowed to open. School children were being taught virtually, along with the colleges and university.

It was during this time that my youngest daughter, Alyssa, was in her last year of university, doing her Bachelor of Commerce, so she had to complete it virtually. This wasn't easy to do. However, everyone got used to the new way of learning. In April 2021, Alyssa graduated. After all the ups and downs, she made it through. Once again, we were very proud of our daughter's accomplishments. She spent many hours studying, and it paid off.

The streets were like a ghost town. Nobody was allowed to be out. The days consisted of keeping up with the news to see what to do next. Every day during the update, there were more and more cases showing up. This went on for a long time. There were all kinds of rules to follow. One such rule was that only one person from a household was allowed to go to the grocery store. This was not going to work for the blind community; most of us need someone to take us places, and handling things is a way for us to know what something is and to help us navigate our way around.

While shopping, people were to follow the arrows and to keep going one way and not to turn back. A person was not supposed to pick up anything they did not intend to buy. This is how strict things became. Eventually, they opened restaurants for takeout, but no one was allowed to eat in.

People were working from home if they could. The only ones who were working elsewhere were the front-line workers. My daughter, Kelsey, was one of them. She was a pharmacist. They were expected to work no matter how many cases of COVID were around, as people depended on them to get the medication and advice they needed. This was a very hard time for our healthcare workers.

Things were even different for businesses that were allowed to open. Everyone had to stay six feet away from each other. This lasted for quite a while. There were times when things tried to get back to some sort of normal, but it didn't last long. There was always some sort of setback. The number of cases would rise, or a new type of the virus would appear. This happened a couple of times. Then, finally, one day the announcement came. It was what everyone was waiting for: someone had come up with a vaccine.

This was a very hard and frustrating time for people who were visually impaired or blind. Things everywhere were strict. People were not allowed to touch things in fear of spreading the virus. This put the blind community in a hard place. Most of us use our hands at one time or another to help get around or see what something is. If we could not do these things, how were we to cope?

Doctors' offices and hospitals were only allowing one person in at a time, so we could not have someone accompany us to an appointment. The threat and fear of this virus was real, and nobody wanted to get it. Therefore, most of us had no other choice but to stay home. Even home was different, especially for someone living alone. They would not get to have contact from family members unless it was by phone or Facetime. There were many who did not know what Facetime was. What were these people to do? They were left feeling isolated and alone. There were many blind people like this. I knew of a couple of people who were blind and lived alone. They both had their own place and for the most part they managed to get through it, but it wasn't easy.

The one good thing that came out of COVID-19 was done by the Canadian Council for the Blind (CCB) in Ontario. They started holding virtual workshops daily. There were times when there would be more than one workshop a day; these consisted of everything from coffee time to learning how to use a new piece of technology. This was very welcoming. It gave people something to do and took their minds off what was going on outside their door, all while gaining knowledge about something new. For a long while, this was the only way to interact with family and friends. It could not be done in person for fear of getting sick.

My bookkeeping business was almost down to nothing, except for the occasional tax return that had to be done before the deadline. This was even hard to do. A person either had to drop off documents outside the door or fax it to us. I didn't know what to do. Nobody was hiring, so I couldn't get a job. How long was this going to last?

Chapter 8:
Setbacks and Breakthroughs

During COVID-19, there wasn't much to do outside the house. I had to come up with some ideas. I started using my treadmill almost every day. I didn't have any trouble getting on it, and I knew the buttons to press to get it to work the way I wanted it to. It was something I became accustomed to. I looked forward to it. I was even losing a few pounds.

Then one day in early summer, when things had settled down, Wally went for a walk with me outside. We only went about two kilometres a day at first, eventually getting up to four. With the little vision I had and my white cane, I was able to follow Wally. This is how we did it. He kept me out of the ditches. Our path would take us over some gravel road and some that was paved. I preferred the pavement. I didn't like the rocks and potholes. We continued to do this every day we could. We even got caught in some scattered rain showers, but someone always showed up to take us home every time. It was good to be able to get out and around in the sun and fresh air. We continued with our walks into the fall.

Then, one day when I was coming out of the store in Carbonear, I felt a pain in my left knee. It was bad; I could hardly walk. I didn't know what I had done with my leg. It hurt so bad all that night. I went to the emergency department in Old Perlican the next day. I wanted to see what was causing the pain in my knee. While there, I saw my family doctor. He checked over my knee, and I had an X-ray done. The X-ray showed I had a mild case of arthritis. It didn't feel very mild. If this was only mild, I didn't want to see it any worse.

For the next week, I had trouble getting around. It hurt to put pressure on my leg. All I could do was to sit around and do nothing. Going upstairs was next to impossible. The pain when I put pressure on my leg was not good. During this time, I was volunteering at Bursey's Convenience and had to take a little time off.

With medication, I eventually started to be able to put my foot to the floor without too much pain; however, it wasn't gone away completely. I decided to go back to volunteering at Bursey's. I was still having trouble getting up and down. Then one morning a couple of weeks later, I was getting ready to go into the store. I was walking upstairs and was almost at the top, when I felt a sharp pain in my right knee. I shouted so loudly Wally came running to see what had happened.

Wally helped me over the rest of the stairs, and I sat down. When I tried to walk, I could not put my foot to the floor because there was too much pain. This meant another trip to the emergency room in Old Perlican. This time I saw another doctor. I explained to him what had happened a few weeks earlier. I was told I had a muscle spasm, and to put a brace or something tight on it for support.

I wrapped my knee at home, but it only made things worse. Something tight wasn't going to work. The next thing I tried was a brace. I kept it on all the time, even when I was just sitting down. I managed to get around slowly, but it was not good. I could not do anything I wanted to. The next time I saw my family doctor, he gave me a needle in my knee to help with the pain. A few days passed, and it wasn't getting much better. I still had pain. I could not straighten my leg in bed. There was no way to get comfortable.

I could not believe it. How could arthritis come on this fast? I thought it just came with a few aches and pains when the weather was bad. I didn't think there would be continuous pain. I did think one day I would probably get it because I had hurt my right knee when I was younger. When Kelsey was young, we went to a fall fair at the hall in Bay de Verde. It was winter, and there was ice on the ground that was covered up with snow. Kelsey and I were walking up to the hall, when we slipped, and I twisted my leg. For the next few days, I had pain in my knee and found it hard to walk. In a couple of days, it got better. However, from then on, I would find aches in it occasionally, but nothing I could not handle.

I was walking every day and thought I was doing well, but apparently, I was not. I was walking too much. My doctor told me what had happened was probably because I had started walking outside on a gravel road with rocks and potholes. Apparently, this, combined with walking up inclines, didn't do any good for my knees.

I was angry and upset. How was I or anyone to know this? If I did, I could have prevented it. I could not see, and now I wasn't able to walk, either. What was I going to do? Here it was only a few weeks until Christmas, and I could not even go to the mall to shop. I had an appointment to get a COVID shot, and it took all I had to be able to walk from the car to the clinic and back.

In early December 2021, I had a vision checkup scheduled with Dr. McNicholas, my ophthalmologist. The first thing done at my appointment was a test on the pressure in my eyes. This was done by his assistant. When I got in to see Dr. McNicholas, he put in the drops as he normally would and looked at my eyes. Then he checked my eye pressure again.

I wondered why he had done this. Afterwards, he told me he wanted to check the eye pressure again because the previous test showed that it was up. This was the first time this had happened since I lost my vision. The second test showed the same thing; my eye pressure was elevated. I wondered what this meant. He then told me I had glaucoma. I was shocked. I could not believe it. What else was going to happen?

This is a question I should not have asked myself, as two days later I found out I had to have a hysterectomy. I had had a dilation and curettage done back in November, the results of which indicated the need for the hysterectomy. The procedure would be scheduled for early in the new year. A few days later, I got the date: January 7, 2022. I spent all Christmas thinking about the surgery. Things like this caused me to be anxious. I could not get it out of my mind.

Just before my surgery, COVID-19 cases had started to rise again, and things were being cancelled. I figured I was going to have to wait. In one way, I wanted the postponement, but in another way, I didn't; I wanted to get it done and over with. When I checked in with my doctor, she told me that there were cancellations, but mine was not one of them. She said it was best for me to have it done now and not to have to wait.

A couple of days later, the surgery was done, and everything went well. I had to stay in hospital overnight and would be released the next day. I could handle this now that the surgery was over. I was relieved to have it done. However, I was still having trouble getting around with the arthritis.

The next morning, I was released. Wally could not even come up to get me. The nurse had to go down with me. I was home for a few days and doing well, when my doctor called me. I was thinking, *What's wrong now? Why is she calling me?* She asked me how I was doing. I told her I was doing well. Then she told me that a nurse on the floor where I stayed had come down with COVID-19, but they did not think I was a close contact. She wanted me to keep an eye out for any symptoms just in case. I could not believe it, but luckily, I did not develop any symptoms. It was a relief.

After all my setbacks, January 2022 went smoothly. Once I was back on my feet after the hysterectomy, I decided it was time to see how I was going to manage my arthritis, I wanted to be able to walk better than I was doing now. Nothing had changed during the past couple of months. I still was finding it hard to walk any distance.

I made an appointment with Frank O'Keefe, a physiotherapist located in Carbonear. I started seeing him in February, and by the middle of March, I was walking a lot better. Each time I visited him he gave me a treatment, and I had to do exercises. He even gave me exercises to do twice a day at home, and he suggested I always wear Crocs around the house. This would help my knees when walking from a carpeted floor to a hardwood one.

At first, I did not think it was going to work, because there didn't seem to be much to the exercises. But I found out that I was doing them wrong, so they were definitely not going to do much for me. Once I got the swing of them, I started to see the difference. I was able to walk farther before my knees would start to hurt. The next step was to get new sneakers. He told me that if I could take a shoe or sneaker and bend it completely in half, it was not good on my feet. I decided it was best for me to invest in a new pair. He once again suggested some types of sneakers that would be suitable for me. I decided on New

Balance and got them at The Running Room in St. John's. I found them a lot better on my feet. I started wearing them all the time.

The next step in my journey to getting around better was to get orthotics for my sneakers. Frank did my measurements and made them for me. When I first tried them in my shoes, I could not believe the difference. They were so comfortable and easy to wear. After a few more sessions with Frank, I was ready to go. I could finally get around. At first, I could not walk or stay on my feet too long, but the more I tried, the better it got. The trick was to not stay on my feet or walk too long when I was having pain. This is when it was time to sit down and relax the muscles. When I felt up to it, I could get up again. The more I did this, the stronger my knees became, and the farther I could walk before needing to rest.

It felt wonderful to be able to get around to do things again. My knees were not the same as they were before all this happened, but by watching it and not doing too much at once, I would be okay. Frank suggested walking for ten minutes every other day to get my strength back.

Outside of knitting, volunteering, and going to bingo, I spent most of my time looking for work. Yes, I went to bingo. A friend of mine, Gladys, would play my cards for me. We went every week. Sometimes we won, and sometimes we didn't, but we kept on going each week. I guess you could say we were suckers for punishment, playing and not winning. I was very grateful to have someone to go with, and especially to play my cards for me. It got me out of the house; I wanted to get out and mix with people.

Next, I joined the Canadian Council on Rehabilitation and Work to help me find employment. The CCRW is an organization that offers many services and programs. They try to match people with disabilities with inclusive employers. CCRW provide direct access to talented and motivated job seekers and in turn building more disability confident employers. Each week, I would have to make a log of the jobs I applied for and send them to CCRW. Their training coaches would then work closely with job seekers and employers to see if they can match a person to a position. If a person wants to continue their education, they can even set them up to upgrade or learn new skills. No matter what it is a person needs, CCRW can help.

I had applied for many jobs, but with no luck. I didn't hear anything back from any of them. I didn't even get an interview. It was very disappointing. I wanted to work, but once again, even with the help of the CCRW, no one wanted to hire me.

Chapter 9:
Getting the Job I Want

A year earlier, I had applied for a job with Revenue Canada, though I figured they wouldn't hire me, and I never heard anything back. Then one day, this changed. I received a notification that they wanted me to do the Korn Ferry assessment. These assessments include a set of exams designed to assess the suitability of candidates and employees for a specific position by evaluating their skills and characteristics.

I could not believe it. They had chosen me. Now I had to find out if I could get the accommodations to do the test. I had found out that the website wasn't completely accessible, so I wasn't going to be able to do the assessment online. Once I found the right person, I reached out to them. When the necessary documents were completed, they would send them to me to sign. Once they were signed and returned, the documents would be submitted.

It took a while to get things in place. But finally, I was approved. I was to do the assessment over the phone with a person handling the accommodations. There were two parts to the assessment, so I did it over two different times. People had told me that these tests were hard, and I did not know what to expect. I made it through both tests, and then I had to wait for the results. It was a nerve-racking time, waiting to see how I had done. However, the day finally came, and I had passed. Once again, I was excited to have gotten this far.

There were other things I was required to do over the next few months. Each time, I had to put in the request for accommodations and wait to get it back. I didn't understand why I had to keep putting in another request, as I had already been approved. They now knew why I needed the accommodations. I had disclosed my disability. In June 2022, I finally got an interview. However, once again this could not be done without the necessary accommodations. Part of the interview included going online and answering questions. For this part, I was given extra time. I got through the questions and the interview. I now had to wait to see if I would be hired.

Time went by, and I still had not heard anything; I was now starting to think I didn't get the job. That is until one day in early October 2022: I got the call, and they wanted me to start the next week! I was to go to St. John's to pick up the equipment.

Wally and I left for the city the next day. Once I got there, the first thing I had to do was to have my picture taken for my ID card. There were several other people there at the same time to pick up their equipment. We all had to go into this room with several desks. This is where we had to sit. Once everyone was settled, they started explaining how to use the laptop and access its programs. This was a frustrating time for me. I could not use the laptop, as it did not have a screen reader on it. I had to get someone else to take the notes for me. I then realized that this wasn't going to work either, as I would not be able to read what they had written. They went through everything, and then I went home.

The training was to start the next day. We had to sign in on the laptop and connect with the rest of our group. I could not take part in this, as my laptop was not made accessible for me. I didn't know what to do. I had to reach out to my team leader to see what he thought. I told him I didn't have the screen reader I needed. He told me he would check things out for me. When he got back, he told me my screen reader had to be ordered in. Now I had to wait because there was nothing I could do.

Day after day went by, and the screen reader did not come in. They gave me a short tax course to do online on my own computer, but this did not take long for me to complete. I was again left waiting, with nothing to do. Then early in November, the screen reader came in, and I had to go to the city to have it installed. This took over three hours to do. I then returned home.

Here I was back home with my screen reader installed and hoping to get on with the training. The first thing I had to do was several tests. This was required for all new employees. The problem was they were not completely accessible, so they had to get another person who was also visually impaired and working with CRA to help me. We made it through most of the tests, but not without bumps in the road. I was now ready to get on with the training, or so I thought.

It was now early in December. They had tried one-on-one training with me, but this still didn't work. They had no idea whether or not the programs I was to use were accessible with the screen reader. Then on a Thursday, my team leader reached out to me and told me they wanted me to go to the city and go in office for a few days to see how my screen reader would work with their programs. I didn't really want to go, but I figured it was the only way to get things worked out. So, Wally and I went to the city on Sunday to stay with our girls.

Monday morning, I got ready and left for the office on the Go Bus. I went into the office and got set up. They had a coach ready for me. We started in on one of the modules. This is what we continued working on for the rest of the week. At the end of this time, my team leader came and told me that the following week, I would be getting a new coach. So, the next week, I continued working on the first module with her. There still had not been any mention of looking at the programs, which I thought was the reason I was asked to go into the office. The next week was a short one because of Christmas and my coach had taken it off, but they would not allow me to also take it off. Therefore, I ended up with yet another coach. It got to be frustrating. Everyone has their own way of teaching and my coach had been changed three times. How could a person learn this way?

After the new year the second coach I was given was back. We continued working on the modules, with no mention of the programs yet. By this time, I was given a new team leader. I kept asking my coach when I was going to be able to go back home to work, and she could not tell me. She just said it would be after I had completed all the modules. I could not believe it. I thought I was in there to check on the accessibility of the programs, and now they wanted me to complete all the modules before I returned home.

It was now February, and I was still working on the modules. If we came to a section where we needed a program, we would just skip over it. My coach said we would come back to it when the program was working. We did this several times throughout all of the modules. At first it didn't bother me, but the further we got along, the harder it became.

We continued to work this way. Now it was March, and finally someone was trying to do something with the programs. We would start to use one program, get so far, and then run into trouble. We had to reach out to IT for help. We would then have to wait to see if something could be done to fix it. This went on for most all the programs; they were just not made to be completely accessible. Once again, it frustrated me. How was I to learn to do something when the program was not accessible?

We then reached out for the help of another employee who was also visually impaired. He told us ways to navigate through certain programs, but it was ways he had figured out on how to get something done. He didn't use keyboard shortcuts; his method was tab, tab, tabbing several times to get where he wanted to go and then doing the same to get back to where he came from. This was great for him, and he had taken it upon himself to learn to navigate the programs. I did not find this helpful; it took too long to get to where a person wanted to go and back again. If it was accessible, all I would have to do was simply press a couple of keys to take me where I wanted to go.

Myself, my coach, and my team leader agreed that the programs had to be made more accessible, so we decided we should contact the CNIB to see if they could help. Jason from CNIB had said he could come in and see if there was something he could do. However, when we asked my manager, she turned it down and said he could not come in for security reasons. The problem remained unsolved.

My coach and I continued with the modules. Finally, we came to the end of them. The next step was to practice some calls. At first, my coach would take them, and I would listen in and ask any questions I had. After doing this for a while, we started on mock calls. My coach would call me and pretend to be a taxpayer, and I would have to find the answers she was looking for. We did this for a while, and I would look for the answers at my own speed and ask questions if I had any. Sometimes it took most of the day to find the answers, but no one said anything about the time it was taking. I thought this was what I was supposed to do. After all, there was a lot of information a person had to go through to find the answers and not having shortcuts to use was taking longer. It wasn't like I could click, click, click and I would be where I wanted to get.

We continued doing this and still nothing was said. I even started to second guess myself. I would ask my coach and team leader if they thought I would ever get it, and they would say, "Yes, you will get it when you get on the phone. Everyone is the same the first time."

It was now April, and it was getting close to the end of my contract. I still had not been given the opportunity to try out the phone. Even my coach thought it was strange that they hadn't wanted me to get on the phone by now. So, what was going on? Why was I not getting the opportunity to get on the phone? One day, there was a meeting, and they wanted everyone on the floor—that is, on the phones—even the coaches. Now I was going to lose my coach.

They wanted me to stay home on Monday and Tuesday and do some self-study. Wally was happy to hear this, as it meant we got to stay home longer. I did this for a couple of weeks. The next thing I knew, we were on strike; it started Wednesday night when I had returned to town. The first few days of the strike I spent making signs at the rec centre. This is where employees who could not go on the picket line had to go. At the end of the first week, I was asked if I wanted to go home and work from there. I was happy to. I continued to work for the union from home until the strike was over.

It was early in May when the strike ended. I went back into the office to continue my training. Once again, I was not put on the phone; my coach and I continued to do mock calls. Nobody was telling me anything. The next thing we knew a meeting was called and extensions were being given, until the end of June. I figured I would get one, and then I would get a chance on the phone. However, my team leader told me that my manager would have to have a meeting to discuss what they were going to do. She did say it was possible that they would put me in a different position. It was Friday, and my contract was to end the following Wednesday. My team leader told me that there should be a decision as to whether or not I got the extension by Tuesday, and she would let me know.

The next week I waited to hear back from her and hadn't, so I left to go back to town so I would be in the office on Wednesday. I had only been gone from the house about half an hour when my cell phone rang. It was my team leader. She said she tried to contact me before I left but could not get me. She then told me I did not get the extension, and I was not going to be put in the rehire pool. There was no explanation given to me as to why they decided this.

I was shocked and disappointed. She told me that my equipment was to be returned the next day. As I did not have all of it with me, Wally turned around and went back to get it. After supper, we went back to the city, and on Wednesday morning, I returned my equipment.

Chapter 10:
Unemployed Again

Well, here I am, unemployed again. I can't seem to catch a break. I find a job, but it is only for a short time. Does it have anything to do with my vision loss? So, what do I do now? I am not going to give up.

One thing I learned while working for Revenue Canada was that I preferred to work part-time, though if the right job came along, I would consider taking a full-time position. While I was working full-time, I didn't have time for much of anything else. I was enjoying being able to get out and socialize with people. However, I could not keep up with my self-care or many other things. I found it difficult to get appointments on the weekends. Everything I wanted or had to do wasn't open. I found it hard to take care of things outside work when working full-time, however this is not to say that I would not take another full-time job. I am still not giving up on finding work. I am currently working with CCRW to try and find something to do.

Since finishing my contract with Revenue Canada, I have been working with CCRW. They are helping me to figure out what it is I want to do now. What are my next steps? Do I want to continue looking for work, or maybe even continue my education? Right now, I am looking at both. I have applied to several positions that are available in my area, including one offered by Opening Doors. This is a program where employers who are looking to hire can post a job, and these positions are then filled by people with disabilities. The candidate who best meets the qualifications for the job and then demonstrates this in the interview is offered the job.

I have been feeling less confident in myself lately, though. It is not something I really considered before, but now I do. Maybe it has to do with the way I was treated and let go by Revenue Canada. It makes me wonder if I can do the job. I am questioning myself.

For the past couple of years now, I have been doing meditation. After coping with anxiety and depression since a young age, I found that meditation is good for me. It relaxes a person and puts them in a different mindset. However, this is not just a one-time thing; it's a lifetime commitment.

During my time in the city, I wasn't as dedicated to it as I should have been. By not meditating on a regular basis, it threw me off. I am now back on track with it. Meditation is something that should be done every day to feel its effects. A person must keep up with meditating because it has to do with training the mind to be more in the moment and mindful. It works to train the brain.

Through meditation, I came to realize some things I wanted to do with my life. One was to write this book and tell my story of my vision loss. A good friend would tell me every time she saw me that I should not let it go. I needed to tell my story. So, after much consideration, I decided it was something I wanted to accomplish. I am not an author, but I wanted to give it a try. If you are reading this book now, you know how it turned out.

I also learned that I want to help people, especially the blind and visually impaired. After living in the city for six months, I realized all the things that are offered by CNIB. I live in a small community, where there is nothing for people like me to do or take part in. People cannot afford to be going to the city all the time to participate in these events, even though they may want to.

Another reason is that people don't always have the transportation. Therefore, I decided it was time to see if this could be changed. So, along with the CNIB, I tried to form such a group for the Trinity Conception area. I had a list of clients from the CNIB, and I called to see who would be interested in such a group.

My search for people looking to join a group has turned out very well. As of now, there are about twenty-nine members. We had our first social at the Harbour Grace hotel. We enjoyed a lunch, and staff members from the CNIB office in St. John's came out and brought out items from the store. There were different types of technology that could be used by a blind person. We are going to plan another event soon.

I hope this group continues, as I think it is something we need. Just to be able to get out and socialize with each other. People are excited to be part of something and have things to do. CNIB in town are always having events and other things for their clients. Together we can help each other.

One other thing I realized I want to do is to learn to play the guitar. One day while listening to the radio going to Carbonear, they were asking the public what course they would take if they could go back to school. There were different answers, and this got me to thinking. At first, I thought it would be math, but I had already done a lot of math with accounting. Then it came to me: I often thought what it would be like to play guitar. I always liked the sound of the instrument but never thought of taking lessons. After all, music is in the blood in my family.

While in school, I played the recorder and ukulele, but this is as far as it went. Guitar wasn't offered at this time, and I don't know if I would have been interested if it was. This is something I think I will really enjoy doing. I just have to figure out how to make it work for me.

I started guitar lessons, and it went well. The instructor wanted me to start on the ukulele; he told me this is what many people do now, as it is easier for someone starting out. However, I wasn't using the ukulele for very long. One day he got me to try the guitar, and both he and I agreed it was better for me. As I was unable to read music, I usually played from memory. I memorized the areas in a song where I had to change chords. I just had to learn the words to more songs.

Chapter 11:
More Setbacks

I continued with my guitar lessons and was doing okay. Then early in November, my dad became sick. At first, we just thought he had the flu. He had gone to emergency in Old Perlican and had a COVID test done. He was sent home, as at that time, it took a few days to receive results. At home, he got sicker. He was having trouble breathing. All I could do for him was drop off food, as we did not know if it was COVID or not. I had to stay away, and instead I would call to check on him every day.

Dad wasn't getting any better. He was now staying in bed all day and not eating. He went to the hospital on Thursday, and when I spoke to him on Tuesday, he had gotten worse. I finally convinced him he had to go back to the hospital. He said to me, "How am I going to get home if they let me out?"

I said, "If they let you out, we will get you home. You don't have to worry about that." I told him to get ready, and I called the ambulance. I also called the hospital, and the doctor on call told me that they had the results of his test, and he had a bad case of COVID. The ambulance came for him and took him to the hospital to check him out, then he was transferred to the hospital in Carbonear.

Dad spent the next two weeks in hospital. He developed pneumonia and was in the ICU for about a week. It was also a week before I was able to get in to see him. I called the hospital two or three times a day to see how he was doing. They were having trouble getting his oxygen level up.

Finally, I was able to see him. He was able to talk, but it took a lot out of him. When I went up again the next day, he was talking better. I thought to myself, *He is going to be okay*. However, his oxygen level still wasn't going up. Then one day the nurse told me that it was up to 98 percent. I thought this was great. He was going to come out of it. Then a couple of days later, I was up to see him, and it seemed like he had gotten worse. I think he was in pain at this time. I heard him make a "grunt" and asked him if he had pain, but he said nothing. He did, however, say to me, "I won't be getting out of here tomorrow," and I thought this strange. I could not understand it. The next morning, I got a call from the nurse telling me that Dad was agitated, saying he was done and that he wanted to see me.

Wally and I got ready and went up to see what was going on. By the time I got there, he was not responding to my voice. I don't know if he was sedated or just unresponsive. His doctor was gone away and there was another one in his place. I told the nurse I wanted to speak to him. When he came up, he asked me what I knew about my dad. I told him I knew he had COVID and then got pneumonia. He told me that several of Dad's organs were failing.

I knew Dad did not want to be put on life support, so where did this leave us? The doctor told me I had two options; I didn't know what to do. I went home to think, though I wasn't home for long, when the nurse called and said that he had taken a turn for the worse.

Wally and I left to once again go to the hospital; however, by the time we got there, Dad was gone.

I didn't know what to think; my dad was gone. What was I going to do now? He was eighty-one, and I knew anything could happen at any time, but I did not expect it to be like this. For his age, he was well and still active. He would go shopping for his groceries by himself. He still had his licence.

My brother Shawn was in hospital during this time, getting treatments for a mental health issue. He was not doing well, and now dad was gone. It wasn't a good time for me. I had to tell Dad's brother, Linus, and sister, Nita. I had been in contact with both since Dad went into hospital. My cousin, Tony, was a great help. I would reach out to him when I needed something. They were all shocked; they could not believe he was gone.

The next few days were hard on all of us. I got everything ready for his funeral with help from my aunt, uncle, cousins, and a great friend, Gladys Sparkes, who went with me to pick out the casket. My brother made it to the funeral. Our father had passed away on November twenty-seventh, and his funeral was on December first. My brother's fiftieth birthday was the next day.

I was getting through it day by day, doing what needed to be done. Then about two weeks later, I woke up and had no feeling in my right arm; I could not even lift it. My right leg was not much better. I had to go to emergency. After some tests, I was told I had had a mini stroke. I wondered what else was going to happen.

The following Tuesday, I had to go to town for an ultrasound on my neck. They wanted to see if there were any blockages. It took close to a week before I started to feel my arm getting better. I would push myself to try to get some life back into it. Eventually, it did come back, but

I still find a little something with two of my fingers. I had to stop my guitar lessons until I saw what was going to happen. The ultrasound on my neck did not show any blockages, and I was grateful for this.

Chapter 12:
Moving On

Well, here I was trying to get back to some sort of normal. I found Christmas very difficult. I don't really know how I was feeling; it just wasn't the same without Dad. He would be up for supper every year since Mom passed away. The girls were out, and Shawn came up, but it still wasn't the same. We had to get used to the new normal.

Since Mom passed away, I did everything I could to help Dad. If he needed something, he would call me. Every night around the same time, I would call to see what he was doing, and when I didn't call, I went down to see him. He lived just down the road from me. He knew when we went somewhere, as he could see from his living room window, where he sat most of the time. When Wally and I drove by, I would ask him if Dad was home, or if he was out by the door. This got to be a habit whenever we went somewhere. I guess I was just checking on him. Now that he is gone, I still feel like doing the same thing, only then I remember he is not there. It's going to take some getting used to. I don't know what it is, but it seems different than when Mom passed away. There are still nights when I forget myself and think I must call him. It was part of my routine.

It was the new year, and I still had not found any work. I had a couple of interviews before Christmas but didn't get anything. I am still looking, but there is not much available in my area. I have been feeling a little depressed since some time before Christmas. I am thinking it has to do with my being let go from Revenue Canada, and then Dad's passing. It's not that I don't want to do anything; it's the opposite. I really want to get out and go to work. All I usually do is go for the occasional appointment or for groceries, which is good, but I want something more. My friends are working and don't have time to get together. I spend my days home wondering what to do. Wally and Nellie go about their business and go to work, and I would not expect them to do any different. I just want to have a reason to get out of the house.

For the past few months, I have been noticing my vision changing, and not for the better. I can't see the sun like I did, and it is harder to find my way around. I can't pick out the food I have on my plate like I used to. I thought it was difficult when I first lost my vision, but now with these changes, it is getting harder. Even though I was considered legally blind before, I could see enough to do many things; this is no longer the case. I don't know if it has to do with my glaucoma, or just the changes due to my damaged optic nerves.

I used to see my ophthalmologist on a regular basis, but since July 2023, this has changed. Before my last appointment, I had a call from his secretary to cancel. She told me that he was off on medical leave and did not know when or if he would be back. She suggested I find a new ophthalmologist. I have been looking for one, but with no luck. I have asked my family doctor and an optometrist, but they have not been able to find one either. It is very frustrating. Here I want to try to keep the little vision I have, but I can't get in to see an ophthalmologist; what am I to do? They seem to have all the patients they are taking on, so where does this leave the rest of us?

Living in such a small area outside the city doesn't offer much to do, and it is even worse for people who are visually impaired or have other disabilities. This is something that needs to be changed. Who knows; maybe this will be my next challenge.

I have decided to put my guitar lessons on hold for now, as Wally is going to work and won't be able to take me there. I haven't gotten my CNIB group together since late in November, just before dad passed away. We had a kitchen party at the Knights of Columbus in Carbonear. I had my Uncle Linus and cousin Tony play for us. The turnout was very good, considering that morning we had snow. Everyone had a wonderful time. My plan is to have a Corn Hole tournament next. This is something new that is growing in popularity. It's like a bean bag toss, where a person tries to get the bean bag into the hole. There are four people on a team. I think this is something that could work. We could have a team with two visually impaired people along with two people with sight.

I will not abandon hope on finding a job. I am going to keep looking. As you should know from reading this book, I am not one to give up. I am going to continue to reach for those stars. I have spent many hours focusing my time on this book, but it has been worth it. Sharing my experiences as a visually impaired person trying to find work will hopefully be able to help someone else and maybe make changes for us in the future.

Chapter 13:
From Darkness Toward Light

It's like I have been on an emotional roller coaster since losing my vision, from trying to find work and everything I have gone through with my family members since. It can take a toll on a person. It doesn't make any existing anxiety and depression better, that's for sure. I had to do something to take back my life.

No, seeing the light does not mean that my vision came back. The light refers to my attitude, feelings and outlook I have found through coaching. The journey to the light is about a shift in how I perceive and interact with the world around me. It's something I work on every day.

For a long time, I harboured anger and resentment. I blamed doctors for my condition, after all it was their negligence that caused my vision loss in the first place. It's not an easy thing to accept, knowing that it could have possibly been prevented. However, by being angry and holding onto blame it became a heavy burden for me to carry, anchoring me in a place of darkness and negativity. The more I dwelled on it, the more it consumed me, turning into a relentless storm of bitterness that overshadowed my life and any possibility of peace.

It took time, but in sharing during my coaching sessions I began to understand that holding onto this anger was only hurting me and nobody else. My rage did nothing to change the past or improve the present; it only kept me stuck in one place. I know now how much better it feels to let it go and move on. Realizing this was the first step towards my healing. This did not happen overnight; it took time and work. I learned techniques to improve my mood and minimize anxious thoughts. I discovered the power of mindfulness and the importance of staying present. Breathing exercises, positive affirmations and gratitude practices became a part of my daily routine.

At first, I wasn't convinced that breath work would do anything for me but once I got the hang of it, I could not believe how it made me feel. It got me through my father's passing and his funeral. I now use it daily. I also began using meditation apps and reading some self-help books which helped me look at things differently. Staying positive can improve not only your mind, but also your body. One such book was *Anxiety Rx* by Russell Kennedy, MD. This book gave me a new insight into what anxiety really is—not just a mental condition, but one that affects the body as well. I found it so impactful that I am currently reading it for a second time.

There have been many things that have contributed to my healing. The CNIB support has been so helpful to me, knowing that there are vision mates and just people to talk to are encouraging. All a person must do is reach out to them and they will help in any way that they can. A vision mate is a person who volunteers their time to help clients of the CNIB who are blind or visually impaired. They can aid in anything from going for a walk, going shopping, going to get a coffee, or just meeting up to have a friendly chat. The CNIB is always searching for vision mates, so if this is something that appeals to you, reach out to your local CNIB office. It will change the life of a blind person. They also have counselors and many other people who understand the struggles that I faced with accessibility. If it were not for the CNIB, I would not have been able to do many of the things I do today.

There are some other things that I have been taking part in, in addition to my CNIB support and regular coaching sessions. I practice daily meditation, avail of massage therapy, manicures and pedicures, reiki and more recently, yoga. These are all ways I offer myself love and create inner peace. I am getting assistance with healthier eating and learning other tools to assist with menopause and anxiety. I am completing a program which involves "chakra clearing" to help express and release emotions and reconnect with myself on a deeper level. I am doing many things for myself and learning to listen to my body.

I am still working on forgiveness; it doesn't matter that I have not reached it yet. It will come in time. It's my intention to get there. Not just to forgive the doctors responsible, but to forgive myself as well. You may ask what did I do? I have to forgive myself for the moments of despair and for the times I let my condition define me. Hanging onto this feeling was only hurting myself. I had to accept that they are all part of me and my experience. This forgiveness is a very gradual process, like slowly peeling away the layers of an onion to reveal the light surface beneath. I am not fully emotionally healed, nor have I eliminated anxiety and stress. This is a truth I remind myself of daily. It's okay to feel this way, it's okay to seek help and to try different methods until you find what resonates with you. There is no one-size-fits-all solution to healing and growth. Each person's journey is unique, shaped by their experience and needs.

Although my life is far from perfect, how I feel and respond to what happens in life is improving. If you are facing something in your life that is difficult, have faith in yourself regardless of what obstacles you face. If I can do it, so can you. You do not have to face these things alone. Don't be afraid to seek help and explore various options. Many clinical and holistic methods have been helpful for me and can also assist you on your path. Remember, you are not alone, and it is okay to ask for help when you need it. Asking for help is the biggest part of the battle. Once you take this first step, it gets easier from there. Don't give up, you will make it!

Dealing with the stress of vision loss or any disability can be hard, but I will repeat myself once more – you are not alone. There is someone out there waiting to help you, all you must do is reach out. There is nothing to be ashamed of, everyone needs assistance at some point in their life. Do not suffer through things alone. Reach out and get the help you need, you will be glad you did!

Conclusion

Vision loss can be devastating. It can affect a person's life in many ways; however, it doesn't have to hold you back. You can still have a very normal life. There is this phrase I heard, and it stuck with me: "I may not be able to see the stars, but I can still reach for them." I honestly believe this. If you want something bad enough, you will find a way to get it.

My journey with vision loss has taught me many new ways of doing things. I even took on the challenge of going back to school, not knowing what to expect, and I made it; I graduated. You can do it too. Just believe in yourself, and don't let anyone change your mind. It's the successes that make it all worth it.

Vision loss affects people of all ages. Some are born with it, while others lose it later in life. It doesn't matter when it happens; it changes a person's whole life. An estimated 1.5 million people in Canada identify themselves as having some type of vision loss. Another 5.5 million have an eye disease that can cause sight loss. Vision loss is expected to double in the next twenty-five years with Canada's aging population.[7]

But the good news is that regular comprehensive dilated eye exams can help adults aged fifty and older protect their vision by catching eye

---

7   CNIB, "Blindness in Canada."

diseases and conditions early, when they're easier to treat.[8] This is why everyone must do their part to make things accessible for everybody else. In the future, there will be more people depending on accessible services. Some things that can be done to make a home more accessible could include good lighting, improved household organization, embracing contrasting colours, thinking bigger, working with a low vision specialist, and providing moral support.[9]

When a person loses their vision later in life, their independence disappears. The little things you used to do becomes a struggle. You must learn to do everything over again.

For a person who is born without sight, it is still just as hard. The difference is, one must start from the beginning without proper vision, while the other has to learn to do things all over again in a different way when they lose their vision. This is not easy for anyone, but it can be done. One myth about vision loss is that people who are blind cannot do anything. The fact is that we can do the same as a person with sight, we just learn a new way to do it. The different types of technology being developed today are making it easier for the blind community to do many things they once could not.

Vision loss doesn't have to stop a person from living their life the way they want to. Today's technology allows a person to do many things that could not be done before. Every day more and more advancements are made. People with vision loss are becoming what they really want to be, the same as anyone else would.

The first thing you need to do is say to yourself, "I am not going to give up, I am going to find a new way to live my life. I am not going to let my vision loss hold me back." If this is what you want,

---

8   National Eye Institute, "Vision and Aging Resources."

9   Bursack, "How to Make Life Easier and Safer for Seniors with Low Vision."

there is nothing and no one who can stop you from doing it. It may be hard at first, but don't give up; keep going. There will be struggles to get through and barriers to overcome, but in the end, it will be worth it. From experience, I know that learning to do something new or figuring out how to do something gives us a great feeling. It doesn't have to be big; even the simplest things give us great joy.

For those who have vision, don't take it for granted. Take care of your eyes, have regular checkups, and play safe. Make sure you don't do anything that can damage or harm your sight. For people who have an eye condition that may cause them to lose their vision, keep up with the research being done, and don't give up. You must take care of yourself. No one is going to do it for you.

As of now, I still haven't found any work, but I am not going to give up. Every day I am checking the job bank and Indeed. I am also still working with CCRW. Maybe one day I will find the perfect job for me, or I may even consider starting a business of my own again. Who knows; the possibilities are endless. I am going to continue with my guitar lessons and hopefully get the CNIB group together.

Writing this book has been a learning experience for me. Until now, I didn't realize the amount of effort that would go into it. There have been ups and downs, but now I am starting to see the results of my hard work. Many thanks to everyone who took the time to read about my journey. This may be the end of my book, but it is not the end of my journey with vision loss.

Bibliography

Bursack, Carol Bradley. "How to Make Life Easier and Safer for Seniors with Low Vision: 7 Tips for Helping a Visually Impaired Senior." Accessed August 21, 2020. https://www. agingcare.com/articles/making-life-easier-for-older-adults-with-low-vision-177792.htm.

Canadian National Institute for the Blind. "Blindness in Canada." Accessed April 20, 2024. https://www.cnib.ca/en/sight-loss-info/blindness/blindness-canada?region=on. 2.

Government of Canada, Statistics Canada. "Census Profile, 2016 Census Carbonear, Newfoundland and Labrador." Census Profile, 2016 Census - Carbonear, Town [Census subdivision], Newfoundland and Labrador and Newfoundland and Labrador [Province], October 27, 2021. https://www12.statcan.gc.ca/census-recensement/2016/dp-pd/prof/details/page.cfm?Lang=E&Geo1=CSD&Code1=1001370&Geo2=PR&Code2=10&SearchText=Carbonear&SearchType=Begins&SearchPR=01&B1=All&GeoLevel=PR&GeoCode=1001370&TABID=1&type=0.

Government of Newfoundland and Labrador. "Lower Island Cove Profile." Accessed June 16, 2024. https://nl.communityaccounts. ca/profiles.asp?_=vb7En4WVgaauzXNjXA__

Grassnickle, Adam. "Your Mental Health: How Vision Loss Impacts Depression." Accessed January 3, 2023. https:// wcblind.org/2022/10/your-mental-health-how-vision-loss- impactsdepression/#:~:text=Researchers%20estimate%20 that%20between%20a,loses%20confidence%20and%20 self%2Dworth.

Kennedy, Russell. "Anxiety Rx: A New Prescription for Anxiety Relief from the Doctor Who Created It." Morgan James Publishing, 2020.

MacNeil, Jennifer. "Let's Boost the Employment Rate for Canadians with Sight Loss." Accessed April 20, 2024. https://www.cnib.ca/en/news/lets-boost-employment- rate-canadianssightloss?region=on#:~:text=Canada%20 has%20made%20great%20strides,triple%20Canada's%20 general%20unemployment%20rate.

Mayo Clinic. "Multiple Sclerosis." Accessed December 24, 2022. https:// www.mayoclinic.org/diseases-conditions/multiple-sclerosis/ symptoms-causes/syc-20350269#.

National Eye Institute. "Vision and Aging Resources." Accessed April 20, 2024. https://www.nei.nih.gov/learn-about-eye-health/ outreach-resources/vision-and-aging-resources#:~:text= Vision%20and%20aging%20at%20a%20glance&text= Many%20eye%20diseases%20have%20no,they're%20 easier%20to%20treat.

National Multiple Sclerosis Society. "Myelin and Multiple Sclerosis."
Accessed April 20, 2024. https://www.nationalmssociety.org/
What-is-MS/Definition-of-MS/Myelin.